T0340040

Medicine and the Inquisition in the Early Modern World

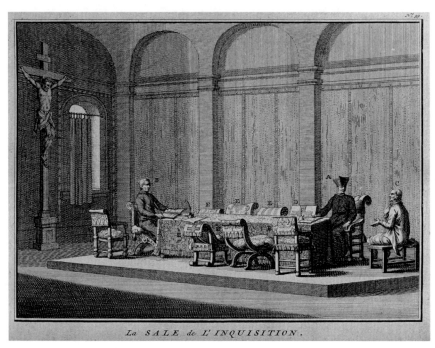

An interrogation room of the Spanish Inquisition with two priests and an accused heretic.
Engraving by Bernard Picart, 1722.

Medicine and the Inquisition in the Early Modern World

Edited by

Maria Pia Donato

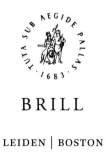

BRILL

LEIDEN | BOSTON

This volume includes the articles originally published in Volume XXIII, Nos. 1-2 (2018) of Brill's journal *Early Science and Medicine* with one additional chapter by Timothy D. Walker and an updated introduction.

Cover illustration: Detail of *An interrogation room of the Spanish Inquisition with two priests and an accused heretic*. Engraving by Bernard Picart, 1722.
CREDIT: WELLCOME COLLECTION, <https://wellcomecollection.org/works/yp9wv5w3>. CC BY 4.0.

The Library of Congress Cataloging-in-Publication Data is available online at http://catalog.loc.gov
LC record available at http://lccn.loc.gov/2019933096

Typeface for the Latin, Greek, and Cyrillic scripts: "Brill". See and download: brill.com/brill-typeface.

ISBN 978-90-04-38645-7 (hardback)
ISBN 978-90-04-38646-4 (e-book)

Contents

Notes on Contributors

Hervé Baudry
is a researcher at the CHAM-Centre for the Humanities at the Universidade Nova de Lisboa, Portugal. His work focuses on the early modern history of medicine and censorship, with special attention to expurgative practices in the areas subjected to the Inquisition. He is the author of numerous studies, including *O livro médico e a censura na primeira modernidade em Portugal* (Lisbon, 2017).

Bradford A. Bouley
is an assistant professor of History at the University of California, Santa Barbara. His research focuses on the histories of religion and science in the early modern, especially Italian, context. His first book, *Pious Postmortems: Anatomy, Sanctity, and the Catholic Church in Early Modern Europe,* was published in 2017. He is currently writing a second book entitled *The Barberini Butchers: Meat, Murder and Warfare in Early Modern Italy,* which will discuss food supply, warfare, and some early episodes in environmental history.

Alessandra Celati
received her PhD in Early Modern History from the University of Pisa in 2016. She is currently a "Marie Curie global fellow" at Stanford University and the University of Verona, Italy. Her research examines the link between sixteenth-century heterodoxy and the rise of modern medicine, exploring the local, national and trans-national levels of this connection. She has published several articles on the reception of the Protestant Reformation in the Italian medical context, and she is currently working on a monograph on physicians and heresy in sixteenth-century Italy.

Maria Pia Donato
is CNRS Research Professor at the Institut d'Histoire Moderne et Contemporaine in Paris, France. Her research focuses on the history of science and medicine in Catholic context and on cultural history. Her publications include *Conflicting Duties: Science, Medicine and Religion in Rome, 1550-1750* (ed. with J. Kraye, 2009); *Sudden Death. Medicine and Religion in Eighteenth-Century Rome* (2014, translation of the original Italian edition of 2010); *Médecine et religion. Compétitions, collaborations, conflits XIIe-XXe siècles* (ed. with al., 2013).

Martha Few

is Professor of History and Gender, Women's, and Sexuality Studies at The Pennsylvania State University. Her work concentrates on the ethnohistory of Indigenous peoples during Spanish colonial rule through the lenses of medicine and public health, gender and sexuality, environmental history, and human-animal studies. Among her publications, *For All of Humanity: Meso-american and Colonial Medicine in Enlightenment Guatemala* (2015). Her current projects include a collaborative monograph on the early history of the cesarean operation for fetal baptism in the Spanish and Portuguese Empires, and an environmental history of insects in the making of the New World.

Guido Giglioni

is Associate Professor of History of Philosophy at the University of Macerata, Italy. His research is focused on the interplay of life and imagination in the early modern science and medicine, on which he has written and edited several contributions. He has authored two books, *Immaginazione e malattia. Saggio su Jan Baptiste van Helmont* (2000) and *Francesco Bacone* (2011).

Andrew Keitt

is an associate professor of History at the University of Alabama at Birmingham. He specializes in the cultural and intellectual history of Spain and is the author of *Inventing the Sacred: Imposture, Inquisition, and the Boundaries of the Supernatural in Golden Age Spain* (2005). He is currently working on a book on the relationship between medicine and politics in nineteenth-century Spain.

Hannah Marcus

is an assistant professor in the Department of the History of Science at Harvard University. Her research focuses on the scientific culture of early modern Europe between 1450 and 1700. She is currently completing a book titled *Forbidden Knowledge: Medicine, Science, and Censorship in Early Modern Italy*.

Timothy D. Walker

is a professor of History at the University of Massachusetts Dartmouth, where he serves on the Executive Board of the Center for Portuguese Studies and Culture, and as graduate faculty for the doctoral program in Luso-Afro-Brazilian Studies and Theory. He was visiting professor at the Universidade Aberta in Lisbon, Portugal, from 1994 to 2003. His research focuses on the circulation of knowledge and healing practices in the early modern, especially Portuguese, world. He is the author of *Doctors, Folk Medicine And The Inquisition: The Repression Of Magical Healing In Portugal During The Enlightenment* (2005).

Medicine and the Inquisition in the Early Modern World: Introduction

Maria Pia Donato

Institut d'Histoire Moderne et Contemporaine, Paris

mpiadonato@gmail.com

Twenty years ago, in an attempt to trace the comparative history of the Spanish, Portuguese and Roman Inquisitions, Francisco Bethencourt noted that the very term 'Inquisition' was foremost associated with the Spanish *Suprema*.[1]

Until recently, the Roman Inquisition appeared to be the least studied of its early modern counterparts. The opening of the archives of the Congregation for the Doctrine of the Faith in the mid-1990s (first to a selected number of scholars, then to historians in general) has changed this situation considerably. Since then, a vast and still growing body of scholarship has shed new light on the Holy Office and the Congregation of the Index of Prohibited Books. The functioning, composition and internal history of both congregations are now better understood, and crucial aspects of their activities have been scrutinised.[2] Comparative and connected approaches, which specialists called for two decades ago, are also ongoing.[3]

Building on such scholarship, a more nuanced appraisal of the action of both congregations has emerged in recent years. Scholars now tend to consider

---

1   Francisco Bethencour, *L'Inquisition à l'époque moderne: Espagne, Italie, Portugal, xve-xixe siècle* (Paris, 1995), 22.

2   Gigliola Fragnito, ed., *Church, Censorship, and Culture in Early Modern Italy* (Cambridge, 2001); Andrea Dal Col, *L'Inquisizione in Italia: Dal xii al xxi secolo* (Milan, 2006); Adriano Prosperi, ed., *Dizionario storico dell'Inquisizione,* 4 vols. (Pisa, 2010); Hermann Schwedt et al., *Prosopographie von Römischer Inquisition und Indexkongregation 1701-1813* (Paderborn, 2010); Thomas F. Mayer, *The Roman Inquisition: A Papal Bureaucracy and its Laws in the Age of Galileo* (Philadelphia, PA, 2013). For an assessment of research trends, see [Accademia nazionale dei Lincei], *A dieci anni dall'apertura dell'archivio della Congregazione per la Dottrina della fede: Storia e archivi dell'Inquisizione* (Rome, 2011) (a second, updated volume is currently in progress).

3   Jean-Pierre Dedieu and René Millar Carvacho, "Entre histoire et mémoire. L'inquisition à l'époque moderne: Dix ans d'historiographie," *Annales esc*, 57 (2002), 349-372; Agostino Borromeo, ed., *L'Inquisizione: Atti del simposio internazionale* (Vatican City, 2003).

them as part of a web of institutions competing to define orthodoxy and to control society and culture. The elusive nature of orthodoxy and the shifting boundaries between theology, philosophy and medicine have been underscored.[4]

Clearly, historians did not await the opening of the central Roman archives to make the Inquisition a historical problem and to use inquisitorial records as a key to accessing early modern societies and cultures. Using local archives and other sources, they have long addressed issues that are at the intersection of religion and medicine, and in which the Inquisition also played a part. Such topics include the verification of sanctity, possession and mental illness, sexuality and gender, birth and dying.[5] Above all, the persecution of magic and witchcraft has sustained, and still does sustain, an inexhaustible body of scholarship.[6]

The predominant focuses for researchers, however, have long been social history and popular culture, whereas learned medicine has remained a secondary subject. In spite of their biases, inquisitorial sources do provide exceptional evidence for investigating lay and popular attitudes towards nature, the body and traditional healing practices.[7] A similar concern permeated scholar-

---

4   Bruno Neveu, *L'Erreur et son juge: Remarques sur les censures doctrinales a l'époque moderne* (Naples, 1993); Susanne Elm, Eric Rebillard and Antonella Romano, eds., *Orthodoxie, christianisme, histoire* (Rome, 2000); Maria Pia Donato, "Les doutes de l'Inquisiteur: Philosophie naturelle, censure et théologie à l'époque moderne," *Annales E.S.S.,* 64 (2009), 15-43.

5   See, in a vast literature, *Cultura popolare in Emilia Romagna: Medicina, erbe e magia* (Milan, 1981); Giovanni Romeo, *Inquisitori, esorcisti e streghe nell'Italia della Controriforma* (Florence, 1990); Anne Jacobson Schutte, *Aspiring Saints: Pretense of Holiness, Inquisition and Gender in the Republic of Venice, 1618-1750* (Baltimore, MD, 2001). Earlier general studies include John Tedeschi, *The Prosecution of Heresy: Collected Studies on the Inquisition in Early Modern Italy* (Binghamton, NY, 1991); on censorship, Antonio Rotondò, "La censura ecclesiastica e la cultura," in Ruggero Romano and Corrado Vivanti, eds., *Storia d'Italia,* vol. v, *I documenti* (Turin, 1973), 1400-1490; Paul F. Grendler, *The Roman Inquisition and the Venetian Press, 1540-1605* (Princeton, NJ, 1977).

6   For a general overview, see Brian P. Levack, ed., *The Oxford Handbook of Witchcraft in Early Modern Europe and Colonial America* (Oxford, 2013).

7   On the theological and cultural biases of inquisitorial sources, see Carlo Ginzburg, *The Night Battles: Witchcraft and Agrarian Cults in the Sixteenth and Seventeenth Centuries* (London, 1983, translated by Anne C. Tedeschi and John Tedeschi from the Italian original *I beneandanti. Stregoneria e culti agrari tra Cinquecento e Seicento,* Turin, 1966) and idem, *The Cheese and the Worms: The World of a 17th-century Miller* (London, 1980, translated by Anne C. Tedeschi and John Tedeschi from the Italian original *Il formaggio e i vermi. Il cosmo di un mugnaio del '500,* Turin, 1976). Ginzburg pointed at the increasing scepticism of inquisitors in relation to witchcraft and popular demonology; nevertheless, the subsiding of the Protestant 'threat' by the end of the sixteenth century led the Inquisition to turn

ship on the Iberian and colonial Inquisitions in the decades spanning roughly from the 1960s to the late 1990s, on the background of post-colonial, subaltern and women's studies.

The opening of the Roman archives made a mass of untapped material available, inspired novel perspectives and sparked new interest for the Inquisition in general, encouraging a return to local sources, which can be now collated and complemented with central records. In this context, medicine has also enjoyed new attention. While some have examined the profile and activities of medical practitioners – surgeons and doctors – who were employed by the Inquisition for the care of prisoners and the supervision of torture, a number of studies revisited the contribution of physicians to debates on those subjects at the intersection between medicine, philosophy and theology.[8]

In fact, the ontological framework that allowed for the Renaissance intellectual encounter between theologians and physicians on demonology, and that informed the Inquisitions' action in the sixteenth and early seventeenth centuries, has been elucidated in classic studies by, among others, Daniel Walker and Stuart Clark.[9] Building on such scholarship, new research has charted the use of medical literature by theologians accurately, tracing the evolution of the inquisitors' 'intellectual toolkit'.[10] It has thus been possible to document how theologians (painfully) coped with the collapse of Artistotelianism and Galenism in framing the preternatural, on the condition that it

---

to other crimes and errors, such as sexual misconduct, witchcraft and unregulated forms of piety. The issue of inquisitors as mediators was also raised by Silvana Seidel Menchi, "Inquisizione come repressione o Inquisizione come mediazione," *Annuario dell'Istituto Italiano per l'età moderna e contemporanea*, 15-16 (1983-84), 53-77. For recent discussions of the shifting perception of magical practices, see Michaela Valente, "Della Porta e l'Inquisizione: Nuovi documenti dell'archivio del Sant'Uffizio," *Bruniana et Campanelliana*, 5 (1999), 415-436; Neil Tarrant, "Giambattista Della Porta and the Roman Inquisition: Censorship and the Definition of Nature's Limits in Sixteenth-Century Italy," *The British Journal for the History of Science*, 46 (2013), 601-625.

8 Federico Barbierato, "Il medico e l'inquisitore: Note su medici e perizie mediche nel tribunale del Sant'Uffizio veneziano fra Sei e Settecento," in Alessandro Pastore and Giovanni Rossi, eds., *Paolo Zacchia alle origini della medicina legale 1584-1659* (Milan, 2008), 266-285.

9 Daniel P. Walker, *Unclean Spirits: Possession and Exorcism in France and England in the Late Sixteenth and Early Seventeenth Centuries* (London, 1981); Stuart Clark, *Thinking with Demons: The Idea of Witchcraft in Early Modern Europe* (Oxford, 1997).

10 Germana Ernst and Guido Giglioni, eds., *I vincoli della natura. Magia e stregoneria nel Rinascimento* (Rome, 2012); Vincenzo Lavenia, "La medicina dei diavoli: Il caso italiano, secoli XVI-XVII," in Maria Pia Donato et al., eds., *Médecine et religion: Compétitions, collaborations, conflits XIIe-XXe siècles* (Rome, 2013), 163-194.

remained Rome's exclusive prerogative to sift through harmless credulity, superstition, imposture or the devil's deeds.[11]

Historians have also delved into physicians' roles as experts and consultants for the Holy Office on cases of possession, simulated sanctity, witchcraft, abortion and generation, sexuality and unconventional healing.[12]

Following archival records closely to trace the physicians' contributions to the inquisitorial machinery – a tendency that is also noticeable for the Spanish and Portuguese Inquisitions, on which a number of insightful studies are available[13] – is particularly rewarding for the history of early modern science, as it enables the scholar to observe with greater insight how the boundaries between the natural and the supernatural, the normal and the pathological, the medical and the religious were negotiated, and how the confines of disciplines were set or infringed upon over time.

Obviously, this shift reflects a more general scholarly interest in the ways in which bodies of doctrines and clusters of concepts were put into action in social contexts, how expert knowledge was translated into practices and, conversely, how practices and contexts shaped learning. This is crucial for

---

11   Elena Brambilla, *Corpi invasi e viaggi dell'anima: Santità, possessione, esorcismo dalla teologia barocca alla medicina illuminista* (Rome, 2010); Fernanda Alfieri, "The Weight of the Brain. The Catholic Church in the Face of Physiology and Phrenology," *Annali dell'Istituto storico italo-germanico in Trento,* 43, 2 (2017), 57-78.

12   See, e.g., Adriano Prosperi, *Dare l'anima: Storia di un infanticidio* (Turin, 2005); Laura J. McGough. "Demons, Nature, or God? Witchcraft Accusations and the French Disease in Early Modern Venice," *Bulletin of the History of Medicine,* 80 (2006), 219-246; Jonathan Seitz, *Witchcraft and Inquisition in Early Modern Venice* (Cambridge, 2011); David Armando, "Spiriti e fluidi: Medicina e religione nei documenti del Sant'Uffizio sul magnetismo animale (1840-1856)," in Donato et al., eds., *Médecine et religion,* 195-226; Vincenzo Lavenia, *Un'eresia indicibile: Crimini contro natura e Inquisizione in età moderna* (Bologna, 2015). Bradford Bouley, *Pious Postmortems: Anatomy, Sanctity, and the Catholic Church in Early Modern Europe* (Philadelphia, PA, 2017). For a later epoch, see Emmanuel Betta, *Animare la vita. Disciplina della nascita tra medicina e morale nell'Ottocento* (Bologna, 2006); Lucia Pozzi, "Catholic Discourse on Sexuality and Medical Knowledge. Changing Perspectives between the Nineteenth and the Twentieth Centuries," *Annali dell'Istituto storico italo-germanico in Trento,* 43, 2 (2017), 95-114.

13   See, e.g., Andrew W. Keitt, *Inventing the Sacred: Imposture, Inquisition, and the Boundaries of the Supernatural in Golden Age Spain* (Leiden, 2005); François Soyer, *Ambiguous Gender in Early Modern Spain and Portugal: Inquisitors, Doctors and the Transgression of Gender Norms* (Leiden, 2012). On the Inquisition's medical staff, see Elvira Cunha de Azevedo Mea, *A Inquisição de Coimbra no século XVI: A instituição, os homens e a sociedade* (Porto, 1997), 469-474; José Pardo-Tomás and Antonio Martínez Vidal, "Victims and Experts: Medical Practitioners and the Spanish Inquisition," in John Woodward and Robert Jütte, eds., *Coping with Sickness: Medicine, Law and Human Rights. Historical Perspectives* (Sheffield, 2000), 11-27.

medicine. As this was an inherently theoretico-practical discipline relying on a casuistic approach, a mildly empirical epistemology and a cumulative method of textual erudition well into the eighteenth century, inquisitorial records provide a good standpoint for expanding our understanding of the intellectual world of early modern physicians.

Last but not least, close analysis of inquisitorial records sheds light on how physicians dealt with their various social roles (e.g., as authors, practitioners, magistrates, men of science, or Catholics) in complying with the ecclesiastical control on society, and the hierarchies of power in which the medical profession was embedded. An essential tension did, in fact, shape their position vis-à-vis the Inquisition: like in other institutions of the sacred, they were caught in the uncomfortable position of affirming their professional autonomy and dignity while acknowledging the pre-eminence of theology and theologians. All this while they participated in the effort to impose conformity.[14]

The changing relationship of mutual reinforcement, alliance or conflict of the Inquisitions and the medical profession is a problem in itself. Across late fifteenth-century Europe, and more decisively in the following two centuries, the consolidation of state apparatuses ran parallel with the strengthening of, on the one hand, corporate institutions, including collegiate bodies for the supervision of medical education and practice, and on the other hand, that of the 'national' Church. However, the balance of power between these institutions varied, as did the prerogatives of the Inquisition depending on the period in which it was created, its structure and evolution, and, most importantly, the political context in which it operated.

Investigating the role of the Inquisition in the repression of popular healing and unlicensed practice under the label of 'magic', Timothy Walker has argued that in eighteenth-century Portugal, academic physicians played a crucial role as part of a global strategy to affirm their control on the market place, which explains why the persecution of folk healers in Portugal increased significantly in that century.[15] In colonial America, the scarcity of medical personnel both left more opportunities for native healers and brought ecclesiastics to the forefront of care for the sick; as a consequence, churchmen encountered the

---

14   On this tension, see Josef Ziegler, "Practitioners and Saints: Medical Men in Canonization Processes in the Thirteenth to Fifteenth Centuries," *Social History of Medicine*, 12 (1999), 191-225; Maria Pia Donato, "Medicina e religione: Percorsi di lettura," in Donato et al., eds., *Médecine et religion*, 11-33.

15   Timothy D. Walker, *Doctors, Folk Medicine and the Inquisition: The Repression of Magical Healing in Portugal during the Enlightenment* (Leiden, 2005). On an earlier period, see José Pedro Paiva, *Bruxaria e superstição num país sem 'caça às bruxas': Portugal 1600-1774* (Lisbon, 1997).

vast catalogue of 'superstitions' embedded in healing practices first-hand, while still forced to deal with medical pluralism.[16]

In Italy too, the Inquisition's action contributed to shape a 'folk culture' distinct (and partly opposed) to the elites'. In the sphere of healing, corporate medical professionals attempted to enforce such distinctions and sanctioned treatments and all other forms of care.[17] Yet it remains unclear to what extent academic practitioners resorted to the Inquisition, or rather operated autonomously in enforcing these boundaries. Possibly because Italy was highly medicalised, with strong collegiate bodies, professional police and social persuasion sufficed to keep unlicensed practice under control. Arguably all forms of therapies, learned, vernacular and sacred, were complementary rather than mutually exclusive in the eyes of the population. Nevertheless, by the early eighteenth century accusations of magic and witchcraft dropped drastically, and even more so the number of trials and convictions. This phenomenon has been credited – at least partly – to the successful rise of learned medicine: although popular healing continued to be used it was discredited to a point that it had lost even the stigma of superstition.[18]

Still, throughout the early modern period and beyond, resistance to the Inquisition remained strong, even among collegiate doctors. As is well known, in Italy the Inquisition was reorganised relatively late (1542), in response to the 'infection' of Protestantism (which, incidentally, spread across all social strata,

---

16   Noemi Quezada, "The Inquisition's Repression of *curanderos*," in Mary Elizabeth Perry and Anne J. Cruz, eds., *Cultural Encounters: The Impact of the Inquisition in Spain and the New World* (Berkeley, CA, 1991), 37-57; Martha Few, *Women who Live Evil Lives: Gender, Religion, and the Politics of Power in Colonial Guatemala* (Austin, TX, 2003); Timothy D. Walker, "The Role and Practices of the Female Folk Healer in the Early Modern Portuguese Atlantic World," in Sarah E. Owens and Jane E. Mangan, eds., *Women of the Iberian Atlantic* (Baton Rouge, LA, 2012), 148-173. On the repression of the use of hallucinogens, see John Chuchiak, *The Inquisition in New Spain, 1536-1820: A Documentary History* (Baltimore, 2012), 308-317; Angélica Morales Sarabia, "The Culture of Peyote: Between Divination and Disease in Early Modern New Spain," in John Slater, Maríaluz López-Terrada and José Pardo-Tomás, eds., *Medical Cultures in the Early Modern Spanish Empire* (Farnham, 2014), 21-39. On traditional (magic) healing, see Laura de Mello e Souza, *O diabo e a Terra de Santa Cruz: Feitiçaria e religiosidade popular no Brasil colonial* (São Paulo, 1986); James E. Sweet, *Domingos Álvares, African Healing, and the Intellectual History in the Atlantic World* (Chapel Hill, 2011); Pablo F. Gomez, *The Experiential Caribbean. Creating Knowledge and Healing in the Early Modern Atlantic* (Chapel Hill, NC, 2017); Hugh Cagle, *Assembling the Tropics: Science and Medicine in Portugal's Empire, 1450-1700* (Cambridge, 2018).

17   David Gentilcore, "Was There a 'Popular Medicine' in Early Modern Europe?" *Folklore*, 115 (2004), 151-166.

18   Oscar di Simplicio, *Autunno della stregoneria: Maleficio e magia nell'Italia moderna* (Bologna, 2005). For a different appraisal, see David Gentilcore, *From Bishop to Witch: The System of the Sacred in Early Modern Terra d'Otranto* (Manchester, 1992).

including medical elites), and on a papal, not a royal, initiative. Although a pontifical 'foreign' institution, it benefitted from the weakness of princely powers and affirmed its prerogatives in a mutually reinforcing arrangement that involved the upper strata of Italian society.[19] But Italy was also the homeland of strong civic traditions and of proud universities prizing their autonomy. Hence, the ecclesiastical authorities had to fight a restless battle against recalcitrant professionals, and a steady flow of literature was produced in order to remind practitioners and their clients that medicine was subordinate to religion. After all, in the eyes of ecclesiastics, physicians were especially suspect because they entered into the most precarious moments of individuals' lives, which could provide the opportunity of inducing them into error, sin and heresy, something for which medical practitioners were sometimes prosecuted themselves.

Indeed, physicians and surgeons were not only experts and torturers for the Inquisition, they were also its victims, and for a variety of reasons. In Spain and Portugal and in their overseas dominions, the possibly foremost reason why medical practitioners faced the Inquisition were their ethnic and religious origins. The Iberian obsession with the purity of blood and the hunt for Jews, crypto-Jews and crypto-Muslims led to an 'ethnic cleansing' of the medical arts at home and in the colonies, and this is arguably another instance of the Inquisitions' regulatory/repressive action in the field of medicine. Notably, the surveillance on Jewish medical practitioners by the Roman Inquisition is a topic worthy of future research, the burgeoning scholarship on the persecution of Jews being one of the most visible results yielded by the opening of the Inquisition's central archives. But in those countries just as in Italy, medical practitioners were also suspect on the grounds of their religious beliefs, for converting others to Lutheranism, as well as for their atheism, blasphemy, the possession of prohibited books and for practising magic, which might include witchcraft and divination. [20]

---

19   Adriano Prosperi, *Tribunali della coscienza: Inquisitori, confessori, missionari* (Turin, 1996); Massimo Firpo, *La presa di potere dell'inquisizione romana (1550-1553)* (Rome-Bari, 2014); Thomas F. Mayer, *The Roman Inquisition on the Stage of Italy, c. 1590-1640* (Philadelphia, PA, 2014).

20   Diego Gracia Guillén, "Judaismo, medicina y 'mentalidad inquisitorial' en la España del siglo XVI," in Angel Alcalà, ed., *Inquisición española y mentalidad inquisitorial* (Barcelona, 1994), 328-352; Richard Palmer, "Physicians and the Inquisition in Sixteenth-Century Venice: The Case of Girolamo Donzellini," in Ole Peter Grell and Andrew Cunningham, eds., *Medicine and the Reformation* (London, 1993), 118-133; Maria Bendita Araújo, "Os médicos portugueses e a Inquisição de Évora," *Universidade(s): História, Memória, Perspectiva*, 4 (1991), 271-280; José Pardo Tomas, *El médico en la palestra: Diego Mateo Zapata (1664-1745) y la ciencia moderna en España* (Cuenca, 2004); Adelina Sarrión Mora, *Médicos e*

True, the loss of most criminal records of the Holy Office, and the fragmentary condition of the records of many universities and collegiate bodies across the Peninsula, leaving aside the lamentable state of many diocesan archives (bishops enforced canon laws on medical practitioners and controlled their morals), makes it difficult to conclusively assess how many medical practitioners were put on trial and why.[21] Nonetheless, regional and monographic studies help to fill the gaps and provide some helpful data on this issue.

It is also true that historians of medicine have scarcely paid attention to the religious roots of the inquisitorial proceedings against medical practitioners, undoubtedly less than the attention paid to the intellectual aspect of what they have long viewed as the eternal struggle for intellectual freedom against obscurantism.

This view dates back to the very origin of (and partially coinciding with) both history of science and medicine, and the history of the Inquisition in the late eighteenth and early nineteenth centuries, when the sacred tribunals were suppressed and their documents partly revealed.

Although the polemics against the sacred tribunals are as old as the institution, the image of the Inquisition as an all-pervasive instrument of control hindering the progress of science and society at large, and as responsible for the decadence of Italian culture, was formulated during the Enlightenment. This narrative was further elaborated within the framework of positivism, which in Italy coincided with the bitter struggle between the newly unified Italian state and the Catholic Church. This legacy helped to shape the Italian national identity from the period of Unification to the present day, and it has had a profound and lasting influence on the history of science and medicine.[22] Likewise, and possibly even more stringently and persistently, a 'black legend' of the Spanish and Portuguese Inquisitions took shape at the turn of the eighteenth and nineteenth centuries, originally fuelled by British and French authors, but soon appropriated by Spanish and later Portuguese national elites in their attempt to

---

inquisición en el siglo XVII (Cuenca, 2006); Federico Barbierato, *Nella stanza dei circoli: Clavicula Salomonis e libri di magia a Venezia nei secoli XVII e XVIII* (Milan, 2012); Jon Arrizabalaga, "The World of Iberian *converso* Practitioners, From Lluís Alcanyís to Isaac Cardoso," in Víctor Navarro and William Eamon, eds., *Más allá de la Leyenda Negra: España y la revolución científica / Beyond the Black Legend: Spain and the Scientific Revolution* (Valencia, 2007), 307-322.

21   Alejandro Cifres, "L'Archivio storico della Congregazione per la dottrina della fede," in [Accademia nazionale dei Lincei], *L'apertura degli archivi del Sant'Uffizio romano* (Rome, 1998), 73-84.

22   Michaela Valente, *Contro l'inquisizione: Il dibattito europeo, secc. XVI-XVIII* (Turin, 2009); Ugo Baldini, ed., *La polemica europea sull'Inquisizione* (Rome, 2015); Massimo Bucciantini, *Campo dei Fiori: Storia di un monumento maledetto* (Turin, 2015).

cope with the modernisation of the state and the supposed backwardness of the Iberian Peninsula and their former colonies.[23]

In all these countries, the persecution of philosophers and physicians for their ideas was a structuring *topos*. One reason was straightforwardly political: many medical professionals were active in the liberal movements and fought against the re-introduction of the Inquisition and the privileges of the Church. Another reason was cultural, for these post-revolutionary liberal physicians-historians failed to fully understand the corporative organisation of medicine and of society altogether, as well as the intertwining of state and Church in the *ancien régime*. These intellectuals therefore disregarded the converging efforts of those institutions to impose social discipline. Last but not least, they tended to salvage some prominent figures from the wreckage of Galenism by making them into innovators thwarted by their conservative opponents, with Galileo as the prime example. These reconstructions globally exaggerated the control exerted by the Inquisitions, while inadvertently contributing to the idea of a 'decadence' of science and learning in seventeenth- and eighteenth-century Southern Europe. Incidentally, the early nineteenth century also witnessed the Romantic recovery of the witch as a positive, inspiring figure pitted against conformism and injustice (including the medical establishment's).

Post-Franco and post-Salazar historiographies engaged in revising such interpretations through a systematic study of primary sources. Censorship of science was addressed through key studies by Virgilio Pinto Crespo, José Pardo Tomas, Israel Révah and others, which put its motives, mechanisms and targets in perspective. While ascertaining the limits of inquisitorial censorship, these scholars nevertheless underscored the culture of control that permeated Iberian early modern and modern societies.[24]

For Italy, too, censorship is certainly one of the areas of research that has most benefitted from the opening of the Roman archives. Thanks to the records of the congregation of the Index and specific series of documents in the Holy Office, like the so-called *censurae librorum*, the effects of censorship on the

---

23   Stephen Haliczer, "La Inquisición como mito y come historia: Su abólicion y el desarrollo de la ideología politica española," in Alcalà, ed., *Inquisición*, 496-517; Navarro and Eamon, eds., *Más allá*.

24   Irvin S. Révah, *La censure inquisitoriale portugaise au XVIe siècle* (Lisbon, 1960); Virgilio Crespo Pinto, *Inquisición y control ideológico en la España del siglo XVI* (Madrid, 1980); José Pardo Tomás, *Ciencia y censura: La Inquisición española y los libros científicos en los siglos XVI y XVII* (Madrid, 1991); Martin Austin Nesvig, *Ideology and Inquisition: The World of the Censors in Early Mexico* (New Haven, CT, 2009); Mathilde Albisson, "Medicina y censura: La literatura médica castellana en los Índices inquisitoriales del siglo XVII," *eHumanista* 39 (2018), 53-64.

fields of natural philosophy and science have been the object of numerous studies and editions of archival materials.[25]

Two main tendencies have thus emerged. On the one hand, some specialists insist on the unrelenting persecution of novel ideas and modern theories by the Inquisition for the sake of scholastic orthodoxy.[26] On the other hand, other scholars point at the regulatory role of the Roman congregations. Elena Brambilla, for instance, has demonstrated the role of the Holy Office in moderating the views on possession and madness through the censorship of handbooks for exorcists. Ugo Baldini has convincingly argued that Roman censorship deprived astrology of social visibility, thus contributing to the disciplinary separation of astronomy and astrology in the seventeenth century.[27] Generally speaking, Baldini argues for a downplaying of the impact of censorship on scientific life in early modern Italy and beyond.[28] Both lines, though contrasting, nonetheless share an approach to censorship as an institution-author relationship, as well as a rather restricted definition of 'modern science.'[29]

Because censorship is now viewed as a fact of early modern societies, the Holy Office and the Index should be understood as regulatory rather than merely repressive bodies, interacting with other institutions of control on a wider scale.[30] Furthermore, as some studies have shown, the complexities of the Inquisition's policies due to its internal composition, and relationships between scholars and men of letters in the Catholic and even Reformed world, need to be taken into account. At a closer look, these factors prove to be crucial in sudden and not-so-sudden shifts in censorial strategies. Finally, the activities of lay consultants and censors reminds us of the obvious fact that no repressive apparatus, however powerful, can operate without some degree of social and ideological acceptance.

---

25   Most notably Ugo Baldini and Leen Spruit, *Catholic Church and Modern Science: Documents from the Archives of the Roman Congregations of the Holy Office and the Index*, vol. I: *The Sixteenth Century* (Rome, 2009).

26   Saverio Ricci, *Inquisitori, censori, filosofi sullo scenario della Controriforma* (Rome, 2008).

27   Brambilla, *Corpi invasi*; Ugo Baldini, "The Roman Inquisition's Condemnation of Astrology: Antecedents, Reasons and Consequences," in Fragnito, ed., *Church, Censorship*, 79-110.

28   Ugo Baldini, "Le congregazioni romane dell'Inquisizione e dell'Indice e le scienze, dal 1542 al 1615," in Accademia nazionale dei Lincei, *L'Inquisizione e gli storici: Un cantiere aperto* (Rome, 2000), 329-364.

29   On this point, see Neil Tarrant, "Censoring Science in Sixteenth-Century Italy: Recent (and not so Recent) Research," *History of Science*, 52 (2014), 1-27.

30   Edoardo Tortarolo, ed., *Censorship in Early Modern Europe*, special issue of *Journal of Modern European History*, 3 (2005); Sarah Mortimer and John Robertson, eds., *The Intellectual Consequences of Religious Heterodoxy 1600-1750* (Leiden, 2012).

And yet it must be noted that in all these studies, medicine has remained a secondary topic, a sub-field of science in general. Until recently little attention was paid to the ways in which the eclecticism of early modern medicine might have informed censorial practices and the strategies for circumventing prohibitions. The typical multi-layered, composite structure of most medical literature of the early modern and modern West, in which several topics and an array of sources and authorities were discussed, made it both easier (depending on the circumstances) to prohibit books, and to expurgate or defend them.[31] The desire to expurgate rather than just censor medical books stemmed from a strong feeling that potentially useful information and knowledge would otherwise be lost. At the same time, because the argumentative style of medical literature was precisely meant to allow expert (and even lay) readers to select and 'pick' what they sought, it also arguably facilitated the introjection of a culture of control – or at least, of a culture of correction, as Anthony Grafton has termed it.[32] Unsurprisingly, physicians working in Rome were especially able in this selective appropriation, though not always safe from evaluation mistakes.

The creative effects of selective reading, of the 'tame' use of prohibited books, and most importantly, of the authors' revisions of their own censored texts are a promising line of investigation.[33] The intellectual consequences of religious heterodoxy also seem to deserve more attention. Keeping in mind the social and epistemic specificities of medicine, future comparative and micro-historical studies of expurgations, auto-censorship, the concession of licenses for reading prohibited books and the market and readership of prohibited medical texts – which many clues suggest to have been extremely widespread – as well as the professional and domestic manuscript culture in medicine will help to rethink the problem of the circulation of medical knowledge in the early modern world.

The aim of this volume is the presentation of new research that specifically addresses anew the role of the Inquisition in various areas of medical theory

---

31   Ian Maclean, *Logic, Signs and Nature: Learned Medicine in the Renaissance* (Cambridge, 2001); Nancy G. Siraisi, *History, Medicine, and the Traditions of Renaissance Learning* (Ann Arbor, MI, 2007); Gianna Pomata, "Sharing Cases: The Observationes in Early Modern Medicine," *Early Science and Medicine,* 15 (2010), 193-236. The argumentative and writing habits of eighteenth-century physicians have not yet attracted the same amount of attention.

32   Anthony Grafton, *The Culture of Correction in Renaissance Europe* (London, 2011).

33   Germana Ernst, "Introduzione: Storia di un testo," in Tommaso Campanella, *L'ateismo trionfato,* ed. Germana Ernst, 2 vols. (Pisa, 2004), 1: VII-LV; Rodolfo Savelli, "Biblioteche professionali e censura ecclesiastica (XVI-XVII sec.)," *Mélanges de l'École française de Rome. Italie et Méditerranée,* 120 (2008), 453-472.

and practice. Each contribution focuses on a specific context or case study while pushing the comparison further between the three Inquisitions. All authors respond to the issues that have been sketched so far; and all argue for the importance of a closer look at the social circumstances for the intellectual history of medicine, as a means of moving forward in assessing the interplay between medicine and the Inquisition.

Hannah Marcus discusses the Roman censorship of medical books and the involvement of physicians in the revision of books on medicine and natural history in the sixteenth and early seventeenth centuries by focusing on a lay censor, doctor Girolamo Rossi from Ravenna. Bradford Bouley considers the use and misuse of post-mortems and anatomical knowledge by the seventeenth-century Holy Office in the definition of sanctity, and discusses the reasons why, despite sharing a similar world view and understanding of natural and supernatural phenomena with learned physicians, the Inquisition did not eventually use medical expert witnesses in many cases. Maria Pia Donato revisits the repression of atheism and freethinking in medical circles at the end of the seventeenth century, and shows how physicians were caught in the shifting balance within the Roman curia.

Moving away fro Rome, Alessandra Celati surveys the rich Inquisition archives in Venice and tracks all the health practitioners that were put on trial in the sixteenth century; she posits that the strong involvement of medical practitioners in the spread of Lutheranism and Anabaptism was rooted in the way they understood their work and their social responsibility for the well-being of their patients. The Inquisition, it turns out, was acutely aware of such sentiments by medical practitioners. Hervé Baudry analyses the manifold activities of the Portuguese Inquisition for 'curing' the 'infection' of heresy and apostasy and the involvement of physicians in such 'cures'; at the same time, however, the Inquisition, supervised the censorship of medical books and the ethnic purity of the medical profession, with a significant number among its victims being New Christian practitioners. Guido Giglioni reconstructs the censorial history of the celebrated *Examen de ingenios para las sciencias* published in 1575 by the Spanish physician Juan Huarte de San Juan. This treatise touched upon the interplay of natural abilities and supernatural gifts, and was put on the Portuguese, Spanish, and later Roman, Indexes; Giglioni examines how Huarte amended his work by engaging with the censors' criticism. Andrew Keitt traces the origins of the myth of the medical martyrs of the Spanish Inquisition in the early nineteenth century: he follows the life of the prominent liberal physician Ildefonso Martínez y Fernández and investigates how Martínez rewrote the story of, precisely, Huarte, in order to advance medical and political reforms.

Enlarging the picture to colonial America, Martha Few engages with the inquisitorial records reporting cases of traditional native treatment for *mollera caída,* a pathological condition in newborns in Spanish Guatemala, and with the question of how inquisitors constructed Mesoamerican medical cultures in terms of practices of the occult such as sorcery, spell casting, superstition; they did not, she argues, attempt to extirpate those practices entirely, but rather to control their inter-ethnic dissemination. In the Portuguese dominions, as Timothy Walker argues in his chapter, there were chronically few licensed Portuguese medical professionals whom the Inquisition could employ for supervising trials. Some cases of medical *familiares* are documented in eighteenth-century Brasil; such men were charged with maintaining vigilance over colonial communities that were considered to be dangerously susceptible to moral and spiritual decadence. In the metropole, though, the intertwining of ecclesiastical and secular elites was so strong that it enabled university-trained physicians to police the professional marketplace through the Inquisition. Drawing upon old and new archival material, Walker provides several examples of physicians and surgeons who worked within the ranks of the Portuguese Inquisition to discredit popular healers in the eighteenth century.

In conclusion, this volume calls for further research in order to advance our understanding of both medicine and the Inquisition in comparative and cross-cultural perspective. Since medicine was at once a trans-regional shared culture with similar institutional patterns, a widely circulating body of learning, and a situated practice and form of knowledge, it seems a particularly appropriate field for addressing this aim.

The Mind of the Censor: Girolamo Rossi, a Physician and Censor for the Congregation of the Index

Hannah Marcus
Harvard University
hmarcus@fas.harvard.edu

Abstract

Girolamo Rossi (1539-1607) was a historian, physician, and prolific censor for the Catholic Church. This article examines Rossi's manuscripts in Ravenna and the Vatican to explore how a physician contributed to the expurgation efforts of the Congregation of the Index in the years following the publication of the Clementine Index (1596). I argue that participating in these censorship efforts trained physicians and other lay experts to read like censors, repurposing the humanist tools of reading, excerpting, and note taking to accomplish the censorship goals of the Counter-Reformation Church.

Keywords

Girolamo Rossi – physician – medicine – censor – censorship – expurgation – reading practices – Index of Prohibited Books – Italy

Censors and inquisitors have recently become a popular and productive area of study for scholars of the Inquisitions in Italy, Spain, and the Spanish Americas. The approach of these studies has often been to break down the congregations of the "Inquisition" or "Index of Prohibited Books" into their constituent

---

* 1 Oxford Street, Science Center, Room 371, Cambridge, MA 02138, USA. I am grateful to Paula Findlen, Maria Pia Donato, the anonymous reviewer, and the participants in the 2016-17 Early Modern Workshop at the Institute for Advanced Study in Princeton, NJ for their comments on early drafts of this chapter.

human actors. This methodology highlights the individual goals and motivations of censors and inquisitors, and challenges the notion that these organizations had agendas and actions apart from the people who participated in them.[1] My study of Girolamo Rossi builds on this approach, but takes as its subject the lay censors who were, occasionally, and for a short time, voluntary participants in the Catholic bureaucracy of censorship. Instead of focusing on professional ecclesiastics, I examine Rossi as a physician and lay professional who volunteered to work as a censor for the Catholic Church.

Formalized lay participation in censorship happened at a particular juncture in Counter-Reformation Italy between the publication of the Clementine Index in 1596 and that of the Roman *Index expurgatorius* of 1607. This expurgatory moment, when the Catholic Church reached out to ecclesiastics and lay professionals across Italy, created a generation of learned readers who read and wrote with censorship in mind. We observe the main character in this study, Girolamo Rossi, publishing books, composing expurgations, censoring his own writing, and ultimately participating in the work of recreating the Catholic Church in the long aftermath of the Reformation by reforming medical and scientific knowledge. Rossi's paper trail is uniquely rich, and can serve as an example to help us understand other pious, Catholic readers for whom the record is less complete.

Despite his well-known importance as a historian of Ravenna, Rossi's career as a physician has never been the subject of sustained scholarly attention, and until Ugo Baldini and Leen Spruit published documents from the archives of the Roman Inquisition, no biographical sketches mentioned his role as a censor for the Congregation of the Index.[2] While learned physicians at Padua

---

1	For a few recent examples see: Ugo Baldini and Leen Spruit, *Catholic Church and Modern Science: Documents From the Archives of the Roman Congregations of the Holy Office and the Index* (Rome, 2009); Martin Austin Nesvig, *Ideology and Inquisition: The World of the Censors in Early Mexico* (New Haven, 2009); Kimberly Lynn, *Between Court and Confessional: The Politics of Spanish Inquisitors* (Cambridge, 2013); Thomas F. Mayer, *The Roman Inquisition: A Papal Bureaucracy and its Laws in the Age of Galileo* (Philadelphia, PA, 2013); and Herman H. Schwedt, Jyri Hasecker, Dominik Höink, Judith Schepers, and Hubert Wolf, *Prosopographie von Römischer Inquisition und Indexkongregation 1701-1813* (Paderborn, 2010). Herman H. Schwedt also wrote a prosopographical introduction to Oscar di Simplicio, *Le lettere della Congregazione del Sant'Ufficio all'inquisitore di Siena, 1581-1721* (Trieste, 2009). For a comparative study of censors that does not deal with inquisition, see Robert Darnton, *Censors at Work: How States Shaped Literature* (New York, NY, 2014). As an earlier example see Paul Grendler, "The 'Tre Savii sopra Eresia' 1547-1605: A Prosopographical Study," *Studi Veneziani*, 3 (1979), 283-340.
2	Baldini and Spruit, *Catholic Church and Modern Science*, vol. 1, t. 4, 2926. On the opening of the Archive of the Congregation for the Doctrine of the Faith, see Anne Jacobson Schutte,

refused to participate in (and even obstructed) the censorship apparatus, Rossi volunteered with enthusiasm. In his story we see a different response to how individuals weighed and balanced personal and intellectual motivations in deciding how they would take part in Catholic Reform.[3] While for some intellectuals these choices led to conflict, for others, like Rossi, expurgatory censorship provided an opportunity for synthesis and accommodation between religious beliefs and medical practice.

Prior to his career as a practicing physician and as a censor of medical books, Girolamo Rossi was a historian, a published author, and a humanist secretary for a famous cleric. The themes of book publication, humanist learning, and devotion to the goals of the Catholic Reformation Church that we see in Rossi's early life remain relevant throughout his long career, which corresponded almost exactly to the period of the most dramatic changes in Roman censorship policy (1559-1607). Through Rossi's story we also trace the continuity of scholarly tools used by physicians between the Renaissance and the Counter-Reformation. The humanist practices of reading and note taking that were essential for learned physicians were adapted and adopted for censorship and book expurgation. The *Index expurgatorius* of 1607, to which Rossi contributed, should be understood not only as a tool for confessionalized reading, but also as an anti-commonplace book. Physicians like Rossi drew upon their humanist educations to repurpose intellectual and didactic tools to serve the Counter-Reformation agenda.[4]

Girolamo Rossi as Historian and Physician

Girolamo Rossi (1539-1607) was born in Ravenna to Isabella Lodovicchia and Francesco Rossi (1503-1574) and was baptized on July 15, 1539.[5] Little is known

---

"Palazzo del Sant'Uffizio: The Opening of the Roman Inquisition's Central Archive," *Perspectives*, 37 (1999), 25-28; and idem, *L'Apertura degli archivi del Sant'Uffizio romano: Roma, 22 Gennaio 1998* (Rome, 1998).

3 This episode in Padua is examined in Saverio Ricci, *Inquisitori, censori, filosofi sullo scenario della contrariforma* (Rome, 2008), 363-376, and in Hannah Marcus, *Banned Books: Medicine, Readers, and Censors in Early Modern Italy, 1559-1664* (Ph.D. diss., Stanford University, 2016), chapter 2.

4 On new Counter-Reformation methods of reading, writing and dissimulation, see Marco Cavarzere, *La prassi della censura nell'Italia del Seicento: Tra repression e mediazione* (Rome, 2011).

5 For basic biographical information on Rossi see Primo Uccellini, *Dizionario storico di Ravenna e di altri luoghi di Romagna* (Ravenna, 1855), 416-417; and Pietro Paolo Ginanni, *Memorie storico-critiche degli scrittori ravennati*, vol. 2 (Faenza, 1769), 313-326.

about Rossi's childhood in Ravenna, though at age fifteen he was taken under the wing of Archbishop Ranuccio Farnese after delivering a Latin oration in honor of the archbishop. Farnese secured a place for the young Girolamo at the Collegio Ancarano, but instead of beginning his studies there, he followed his uncle, Giovan Battista Rossi, to Rome.[6]

Rossi pursued studies at the Sapienza in Rome, under the supervision of Francesco Sempronio and a certain "Bishop Giacomello."[7] He returned to Ravenna in 1560, at the age of twenty-one. The next year he obtained a degree in arts and medicine from the University of Padua. Rossi's eighteenth-century biographer suggests that in 1561, the young graduate returned to Ravenna to begin assembling documents for a book on the history of Ravenna. However, Rossi's career again took an unexpected turn. In 1562, the uncle he had once followed to Rome, Giovan Battista Rossi, was elected Vicar General of the Carmelite Order. Girolamo did not take orders, but he did follow the Vicar General around the Veneto while he visited monasteries, helping his uncle with his public disputations and writing his letters, presumably in the capacity of a secretary. In 1564, Giovan Battista was promoted again, this time to General of the Carmelite Order, and Girolamo once more joined him in Rome.[8]

It was during this second trip to Rome that Girolamo Rossi began working in earnest on the history of Ravenna, for which he would become famous.[9] Rossi began his research for this work in Rome, making use of Roman libraries on his visits to his uncle's monastery. Rossi's early archival research has made his *Historiarum Ravennatum libri decem* among the best known and most widely referenced sources on the history of Ravenna. The Senate of Ravenna paid for the publication of the first edition of the book to be printed by the press of Aldo Manuzio the Younger in 1572 and then paid for the book to be reprinted in 1589 in Venice at the Guerra press, decrying that "one can no longer get a copy, much

---

6   The Collegio Ancarano was among the best schooling opportunities available in Bologna, considered second only to the Collegio di Spagna. Christopher Carlsmith, "'Cacciò fuori un bastone bianco': Conflicts between the Ancarano College and the Episcopal Seminary in Bologna," in Samuel Kline Cohn and Fabrizio Ricciardelli, eds., *The Culture of Violence in Renaissance Italy: Proceedings of the International Conference, Georgetown University at Villa le Balze, 3-4 May, 2010* (Florence, 2012), 194-195.

7   Uccellini, *Dizionario storico*, 416-417.

8   Ginanni, *Memorie*, 314.

9   Eric Cochrane placed Rossi's work in his category of the 'definitive histories' of the 1580s and 1590s. See Eric W. Cochrane, *Historians and Historiography in the Italian Renaissance* (Chicago, IL, 1981), 284-291.

to the disgust of this city."[10] The expertise that Rossi developed as a historian continued to feature in his intellectual life, even as his career shifted toward the study of medicine.[11]

While recent studies of Rossi's work have identified him first and foremost as a physician, little of his career as a doctor has been studied by historians.[12] Yet, Rossi was a well-respected physician; over the course of his life he repeatedly turned down offers of university positions in Ferrara, Bologna, and Rome that would have forced him to leave Ravenna (though the honor of papal physician was eventually too great to refuse).[13] He corresponded with the physicians Ulisse Aldrovandi, Girolamo Mercuriale, Fulvio Angelini, Gasparo Tagliacozzi, Marco degli Oddi, and Arcangelo Piccolomini. He exchanged letters and treatises with two members of the Paduan congregation of censors: Ercole Sassonia and Girolamo Fabrizi d'Acquapendente.[14] Despite his location in Ravenna, Rossi was well connected within the Italian medical republic of letters.[15]

Although there is no evidence that Rossi, like Mercuriale or Aldrovandi, corresponded with Protestant medical colleagues living across the Alps, he was both flattered and worried when his book *On Distillation,* which he had published in Ravenna in 1582 with Francesco Tebaldini, was reprinted without his knowledge in Basel in 1585 by Sebastian Henric Petri, the son of Henricus Petrus. The press, commonly called the Officina Henricpetrina, was famous for having printed a number of books that had been, or would be, banned in Italy, including several editions of Sebastian Münster's *Cosmographia* and the second edition of Nicolaus Copernicus's *De revolutionibus* (1566). Mention of this piracy first appeared in Rossi's correspondence in 1595, and by 1596 Rossi had

---

10 On Rossi's research and sources, see Mario Pierpaoli, "Girolamo Rossi medico e storico ravennate," in Girolamo Rossi, *Storie Ravennati,* ed. Mario Pierpaoli (Ravenna, 1996), XIV-XV.

11 On the relationship between medicine and history writing in this period, see Nancy Siraisi, *History, Medicine, and the Traditions of Renaissance Learning* (Ann Arbor, MI, 2007), and Gianna Pomata and Nancy G. Siraisi, eds., *Historia: Empiricism and Erudition in Early Modern Europe* (Cambridge, MA, 2005).

12 Rossi, *Storie Ravennati,* XIV.

13 Ginanni, *Memorie,* 317.

14 Biblioteca Classense, Ravenna, Italy (hereafter BCRa), Fondo Manoscritti, Manoscritti vari di Girolamo Rossi, Mob. 3. 1 B, n. 1, see ff. 131r, 152r-154v, 156r.

15 For more on the genre of medical epistolary in the sixteenth century, see Nancy Siraisi, *Communities of Learned Experience: Epistolary Medicine in the Renaissance* (Baltimore, MD, 2013), and Ian Maclean, "The Medical Republic of Letters before the Thirty Years War," *Intellectual History Review,* 18 (2008), 15-30.

begun to take steps to have his work printed yet again.[16] The work, a sparsely illustrated, nearly 300-page manual dedicated to Francesco I, the Grand Duke of Tuscany, explained the distillation of liquids and medicines and discussed chemical experiments. The Officina Henricpetrina must have seen an opportunity in this Latin volume to profit from the increasing interest in chemical medicine, especially in Northern Europe.

Because the Basel reprint had occurred without his knowledge or participation, Rossi was intent on having his book republished and wanted to correct errors that he had noticed in the pirated edition. Rossi wrote to Fabio Paolini, the public reader charged with the task of prepublication censorship in Venice, in May 1596:

> I am sending my book *On Distillation*, which was already printed in this city in quarto and reprinted in Basel in octavo, and since the reprint occurred without my knowledge, they were not able to correct some additions that I send now [...]. I greatly desire in any case that it be corrected and that you do not find it unworthy of being reprinted.[17]

Rossi understood the costs and implications of reprinting his book, indicating that he was willing to help finance the publication and that he knew that the format might need to be reduced. Finally, he implored Paolini that the work should be "well corrected," specifying in a postscript that Paolini should "choose among the letters something that isn't too big nor too small, but that suits the page."[18] The pirating of his book by Protestant printers in Basel led Rossi to update his own work, which was published in a new edition in 1599 by Domenico and Giovan Battista Guerra. The work was reprinted yet again in Venice in 1604 by Giovan Battista Ciotti, the printer and bookseller so highly favored by Giordano Bruno.[19] It is clear from the publishing and republishing of his book *On Distillation* that Rossi was also well aware of the paradoxes au-

---

16   BCRa, Mob. 3. 1 B, n. 5, ff. 436r, 443r.

17   Ibid., f. 443r. Letter dated May 18, 1596. "Nondimeno mando un mio libro de Destillatione gia stampato in questa citta in quarto et ristampato in Basilea in ottavo: et perché quella ristampata fu senza mia saputta, non vi potevo aggiungere alcuni additioni che hora mando [...] desidarerei bene che in ogni evento, fosse ben corretto; et che da VS fosse giudicato al tutto non indegno d'esser ristampato."

18   Ibid., f. 458r-v.

19   Massimo Firpo, "Giovanni Battista Ciotti," *DBI*, vol. 25, 692-696. It is also interesting to note that Ciotti was arrested by the Venetian Inquisition in 1599 for importing prohibited books. Paul F. Grendler, *The Roman Inquisition and the Venetian Press, 1540-1605* (Princeton, NJ, 1977), 280.

thors faced when their works crossed confessional divides in Europe. The Protestant, pirated edition of his *On Distillation* simultaneously extended his readership, corrupted his text, and provided the impulse and opportunity to issue new editions of his own. His experience correcting a text originating from Protestant presses, in this case his own book, was in some respects a complementary process to the expurgations that he performed as a censor for the Catholic Church.[20]

Throughout his career as a physician, Girolamo Rossi worked closely with printers and the republic of letters, exchanging correspondence with the major figures on the Italian peninsula ranging from Girolamo Mercuriale and Ulisse Aldrovandi to Paolo Manuzio and Aldo Manuzio the Younger. It is perhaps no surprise, then, that when the expurgatory moment of the late 1590s reached Ravenna, this learned and celebrated scholar volunteered his expertise and intellect to expurgate books. Rossi conducted his research and scholarship with a constant attention to publication and to sharing his ideas with a broad audience in Italy and even across the Alps.

Girolamo Rossi as Censor

Following the publication of the Clementine Index in 1596, bishops formed congregations of censors in cities across the Italian peninsula. One such congregation convened in Faenza under the jurisdiction of the bishop Gian Antonio Grassi. Bishop Grassi received his copy of the Clementine Index and published it in July 1596. On December 21, 1596 he wrote to the Congregation of the Index in Rome that he had "the list of all the books to remove the bad and correct what needs correcting. To that end, I have deputized learned men in all the sciences – that is, theology and philosophy, and canon and civil law, and

---

20   In addition to his history of Ravenna and books on distillation, Rossi published widely on a number of other topics. Among his medical works are a short pamphlet (really a collection of medical letters) about melons and asthma, *Diputatio de melonibus...* (Venice, 1607), and his commentary on Celsus dedicated to Scipione Borghese and published posthumously by his son Francesco, *Annotationes in libros octo Cornelii Celsi...* (Venice, 1616). Rossi exchanged treatises on the plague with Girolamo Mercuriale in the 1570s, which, though not printed, were certainly disseminated in manuscript form. Copies exist among Rossi's own papers BCRa, Ms. 3. 1 B, n. 1, ff. 162r-169v, and in the Biblioteca Ambrosiana, Milan, Italy, Ms. Q. 117 sup. "Miscellaneo," ff. 168r-171v. The Vatican Library also holds an unpublished and likely incomplete work written mostly in Rossi's hand and titled *Rerum naturalium,* BAV, Vat.lat.5361.

the humanities."[21] The Dominican Inquisitor of Romagna, Alberto Chelli, wrote repeatedly from Faenza to the congregation in Rome to update the Congregation of the Index on the progress of his censors.[22] This correspondence is an especially important example of how the censorship efforts connected Rome with intellectual sites around Italy. These congregations also sought to solidify Rome's political interests in a region that was becoming something of a frontier between Venetian interests and the papal state.[23]

Within two weeks of convening the congregation, the Inquisitor of Faenza wrote to report that, "thank God," no one was lacking in diligence in attending to the expurgation of books, some of which were noted in the Index and others of which were not and "had not been observed in the past."[24] We might imagine that Chelli felt some degree of relief, since lay intellectuals in other parts of Italy had not been so eager to comply.[25] Along with the letter, Chelli sent a list of medical books that had been checked and corrected by Giovanni Battista Codronchi, a physician from Imola and a *qualificator*, or outside consultant, for the Index.[26] Codronchi, later himself a priest, was at that time a physician, trained at the University of Bologna and living and working in Imola.[27] Codronchi's expurgations were also undersigned by three other officials of the

---

21   Archive of the Congregation for the Doctrine of the Faith, Vatican City (hereafter ACDF), Index III, vol. I, f. 381r. "Subito che usci fuori il novo indice reformato d'ordine di Nostro Signore il Padre Inquisitore et io publicassimo unitamente editti per la città et Diocesi per haver lista di tutti i libri, per levar li cattivi et corregere quelli che si hanno bisogno, et a tal effetto havemo deputato huomini dotti in tutte le scienze, cosi di Theologia come di Filosofia, et di Canonica et Civile, et di humanita."

22   Fra Alberto Chelli was the inquisitor of Romagna from 1592-1599 and the Inquisitor of Cremona from 1600-1603. Baldini and Spruit, *Catholic Church and Modern Science*, vol. I, t. 4, 2827. For an account of Chelli's arrest and accused conspiracy against Venice see Grendler, *The Roman Inquisition and the Venetian Press*, 216-218.

23   The late 1590s were a particularly key moment for this frontier as Ferrara became part of the Papal State in 1598.

24   ACDF, Index III, vol. III, f. 108v. Also in Baldini and Spruit, *Catholic Church and Modern Science*, vol. 1, t. 1, 619.

25   In fact, many had been obstructionist. Additionally, local congregations charged with correcting books often led to jurisdictional conflict between local bishops and inquisitors. Gigliola Fragnito, "The Central and Peripheral Organisation of Censorship," in Gigliola Fragnito, ed., *Church, Censorship, and Culture in Early Modern Italy* (Cambridge, 2001), 13-49.

26   These expurgations can be found in ACDF, Index, Protocolli, O (II.a.13) ff. 258r-264v, also published in Baldini and Spruit, *Catholic Church and Modern Science*, vol. 1, t. 1, 607-618.

27   Carlo Colombero, "Giovan Battista Codronchi," *DBI*, vol. 26, 604-605; and Luigi Angeli, *Sulla vita e su gli scritti di alcuni medici imolesi: Memorie storiche* (Imola, 1808), 153-169.

local Inquisition: a vicar of the Inquisition in Imola, Michele da Lugo; the Vicar General of the Inquisition in Imola; and the Inquisitor of Romagna, Alberto Chelli.[28]

The congregational approach to censorship outside of Rome relied on input from lay experts in cooperation with inquisition officials. By mid-February the Inquisitor of Faenza had also received expurgations of medical books written by Girolamo Rossi from Ravenna, whom he described to the Congregation of the Index in Rome as "an intelligent physician, and one of those deputized in this city to expurgate medical books."[29] In addition to supplying a list of words and sections to be removed, Rossi also explained why they needed to be expurgated so that no one could accuse him of having "removed them without reason."[30] The expurgations included corrections to three important and regularly requested medical works: the Portuguese crypto-Jew Amatus Lusitanus's *Centuriae*, and the ever-controversial Girolamo Cardano's supplement to the almanac and his astrological commentaries on Ptolemy's *Tetrabiblos* with its notorious geniture of Jesus Christ.[31] Throughout the spring of 1597 Alberto Chelli continued to receive and forward expurgations written by Codronchi and Rossi, but by March 1598 Rossi appears to have by-passed the intermediary of the local inquisitor and sent his expurgations of works by Guglielmo Grataroli and Merlin Cocai directly to Rome. Rossi's letter noted that he was still completing other expurgations, including the works of the infamous physician and religious controversialist Thomas Erastus, which he had already finished making note of but stopped because of other occupations.[32]

Rossi's direct interaction with the congregation in Rome seems not to have been a problem for the inquisitor Chelli or his vicars, who also continued forwarding Rossi's expurgations in the summer of 1599 when Rossi completed further censures of Erastus and Lusitanus.[33] However, in the fall of 1599 Chelli was reassigned to the post of the Inquisitor of Cremona and was replaced by Pietro Martire Rinaldi. On December 3, 1599 Cardinal Agostino Valier wrote to Chelli in his new post to praise the speed with which he had responded to help create the *Index expurgatorius*. Valier suggested further that Chelli could

---

28   Baldini and Spruit, *Catholic Church and Modern Science*, vol. 1, t. 1, 618.

29   ACDF, Index III, vol. III, f. 110r.

30   BCRa, Mob. 3. 1 B, n. 5, f. 448r. Dated 15 February 1597.

31   Lusitanus's *Centuriae* was published in seven installments between 1549 and 1570 and was republished regularly into the seventeenth century. On Cardano's geniture of Jesus, see Anthony Grafton, *Cardano's Cosmos: The Worlds and Works of a Renaissance Astrologer* (Cambridge, MA, 1999), 152, 154-155.

32   BCRa, Mob. 3. 1 B, n. 5, f. 455v. Dated 27 March 1598.

33   ACDF, Index III, vol. IV, ff. 82r-83v, and f. 191r.

"censor some books of medicine or philosophy, or maybe from books of astrology you can chose the ones that can be useful for navigation, agriculture, and medicine, trimming off all that is superfluous and pernicious, and putting together what good there is from one and the other."[34] Careful expurgation, for Valier, was a process through which the Church could salvage the utility of books while curbing the circulation of harmful and heretical ideas. The purpose of expurgation was to preserve knowledge and create books that took advantage of prohibited learning without compromising the Catholic faith. However, when Valier composed this letter to Chelli he had momentarily overlooked the content expertise that had been so essential for Chelli's earlier productivity. The inquisitor was the spiritual authority, but Rossi and Codronchi had been the medical experts who had trimmed from and recompiled the prohibited works that were necessary for Catholic doctors.

While Chelli and his team had been undeniably productive, the new inquisitor Pietro Martire Rinaldi had different priorities for his office. He reported to Rome in August 1600 that the inquisition in Faenza was very busy and could not attend to the correction of books. A separate letter from the Bishop Gian Antonio Grassi in November 1600 confirmed the opposite: a congregation for the correction of books would once again be instituted in Faenza.[35] Perhaps in light of these different agendas Girolamo Rossi began forwarding his expurgations to Rome in the early years of the seventeenth century, often bypassing local intermediaries.

On July 31, 1602 Rossi responded directly to a letter from the Congregation of the Index in Rome, stating that with his letter he was sending the expurgations that he had made "at different times of books of various professions and especially medicine." He continued, "I have collected them into a volume (corpo) [...] and as soon as our Monsigneur Archbishop's new vicar arrives, which should be any day, he said he will review and undersign the expurgations along with the three deputized theologians."[36] Rossi considered this work important enough to have kept copies of these censures among his own treatises and cor-

---

34   Baldini and Spruit, *Catholic Church and Modern Science*, vol. 1, t. 1, 559-560. "In questo mense potrà censurare qualche libro di Medicina, ò Philosofia, [...] ò pur da libri di Astrologia far scelta di quello che può servire alla Nautica, agricoltura, et Medicina, accio si possa resecar tutto il superfluo, è pernitioso, et metter insieme quanto ci è di buono nel uno, et nel altro."

35   ACDF, Index III, vol. V, f. 450r.

36   Ibid., vol. VI, f. 6r-v. "Conforme a quanto Vostro Signore Illustrissima per la sua lettera de li 17 mi comanda, le espurgationi che io ho fatto in diversi tempi di alcuni libri di varie professioni et mass[im]e di medicina, io raccogliere in un corpo, [...] et quanto prima sarà arrivato il nuovo Vicario di Monsignor Arcivescovo Nostro, che s'aspetta in breve, ha detto

respondence.[37] As it turned out, he was wise to have made extra copies. In February 1602, the Vicar, Fabio Tempestivo, anxiously wrote to Rome, expressing surprise that he had never heard back from the congregation about Rossi's expurgations of Cardano, which he had sent a year earlier. "Please let me know," he urged, "because if it was not received I will send another copy, as with this letter I send the correction of the *Scuola salernitana*, done by the same Signor Girolamo Rossi."[38] Writing expurgations required substantial effort, and all parties wanted to ensure that this work would not be lost in transit through early modern postal systems.

Another change of inquisitorial personnel in 1602-03 yet again heralded a reorganization of the Faenza congregation charged with correcting books. On October 24, 1602 the Inquisitor complained that small cities like Faenza could not be expected to produce corrections of books. The "learned men" with whom he had spoken claimed that this task needed to take place in the "big [cities] and the general universities."[39] Turning to the major centers of learning in Italy had, of course, been the Church's original plan. However, that model, which had met with such resistance in places like Padua and Bologna, had since been abandoned. Now communities that were less intellectually central but more reliably productive, like the congregations in Faenza and Naples, had emerged as the main sites of correction. The next August, in 1603, a new Inquisitor of Faenza reported from Imola that in his territories there were not enough people "capable of revising books" to make up a congregation. It is perhaps not a coincidence that the very next day, August 7, 1603, Girolamo Rossi wrote to Rome complaining of the difficulties of working with other people to produce the desired expurgations:

> If the task of sending the censures were only up to me, according to my duty, they already would already be [sent] a long time ago [...] but since it depends on others, I don't know what I can do, except to complete my

---

di fare, insieme con esso lui, la deputatione de li tre Theoolgi che Vostro Signore Illustrissima commanda i quali riveggano et sottoscrivano dette spurgationi."

37 BCRa, Mob. 3. 1 B, n. 3: "Hier Rubei Correctiones 1) in Cardani opuscula 2) in Centurias Amati Lusitani 3) in librum de conservanda bona valetudine Arnoldi Novicomentis."

38 ACDF, Index III vol. VI, f. 7r. "Non havend'havuto mai avviso della recevuta mi son maravigliato, et desidero, che resti servita d'avvisarmene, perché quando non fusse capitata se ne mandarà una copia, si come con questa mia mando la corretione, fatta dall'istesso Signore Gerollamo Rossi sopra la schola Salernitana, che aspettaro d'intender l'habbia recenta."

39 Ibid., vol. V, f. 453r-v.

part of the said service perfectly, copying the censures, and to solicit, as I have already done, those things that the others deal with.[40]

The congregational approach to censorship, in which groups of experts and theologians were convened in different cities and tasked with correction, was fundamentally collaborative and always fraught. While Girolamo Rossi in Ravenna painstakingly expurgated books, his authority derived from his position as part of a congregation of censors, and then that authority was still subservient to that of the Congregation of the Index in Rome.

Rossi persisted at his task in the following months, despite the miscommunication that must have occurred between Rossi in Ravenna and the Holy Office in Faenza. These difficulties with the congregation of censors did not tarnish Rossi's reputation with the curia, however. In 1604 he travelled to Rome as an ambassador, and Pope Clement VIII appointed Rossi papal physician. Rossi's tenure as papal physician coincided with Clement's final months, and the death of the pope on March 5, 1605 brought about Rossi's return to his home in Ravenna.[41]

Rossi composed censures of at least thirteen books, at least twelve of which were sent to the Congregation of the Index in Rome (see Table 1). He provided the Congregation with in-depth descriptions of problematic passages and his reasons for removing them. Rossi's expurgations were primarily of a confessional rather than medical nature.[42] He proposed the removal of passages that mocked the clergy (see Fig. 1), praised non-Catholic scholars, or included citations of Protestant authors. A few expurgations dealt with the intellectual aspects of medicine, considering the influences of God, demons, astrology, and magical words on the human body with respect to sickness and health. Reading carefully with confessional differences in mind was a skill cultivated

---

40   Ibid., vol. VI, f. 11r-v. "Se a me solo stesse il totale compimento di mandare le censure fatte, già molto tempo, conforme al debito mio, sarebbono costì a servire Vostro Signore Illustrissima ma poiché il più depende da altri, io non so che poter fare, salvo che da la parte mia compire perfettamente il detto servitio, copiando le censure, et in quello che a gli altri tocca[?] sollecitare si come ho già anco' hora fatto."

41   Pope Clement VIII had been periodically quite ill for several years when Rossi entered the scene, and he died of a stroke on March 5, 1605. Ludwig von Pastor, *The History of the Popes, From the Close of the Middle Ages* (London, 1906), vol. 24, 430-434.

42   Many of Rossi's expurgations have been published by Baldini and Spruit with some commentary in the notes. See *Catholic Church and Modern Science*, vol. 1, t. 2, 1354-1376, 1390-1404, 1491-1494, 1569-1588, 1889-1893. On the relationship between the natural sciences and the Congregations of the Inquisition and Index, see Maria Pia Donato, "Scienze della natura," in Adriano Prosperi, ed., *Dizionario storico dell'Inquisizione* (Pisa, 2010), 1394-1398.

TABLE 1   *Works expurgated by Girolamo Rossi*

Expurgations submitted in 1597:

- Girolamo Cardano, *De supplemento almanach*
- Girolamo Cardano, *Quadripartitum Ptolomei*
- Girolamo Cardano, *De geniturarum exemplis*
- Conrad Dasypodius, *Quadripartitum Ptolomei*
- Amatus Lusitanus, *Centuriae*

Expurgations submitted in March 1598:

- Guglielmo Grataroli, *Opuscula*
- Merlin Cocai [Teofilo Folengo], *Macaronica*
- [Teofilo Folengo], *Zanitonella sive innamoramentum Zaninae et Tonelli*

Expurgations submitted in February 1599:

- Thomas Erastus, *Disputationes de medicina nova Philippi Paracelsi*
- Thomas Erastus, *De astrologia divinatrice epistola*
- Thomas Erastus, *Disputationes de putredine et de febribus putridis*

Expurgations submitted in 1602:

- Arnald of Villanova, *De conservanda bona valetudine*

Expurgations never submitted:

- Girolamo Cardano, *De subtilitate*

---

through censorship and one which the censor Girolamo Rossi had clearly mastered.

In the end, the vast majority of Rossi's expurgatory efforts were never integrated into the expurgations that Rome eventually published in 1607. A line by line comparison of the censures that he composed reveals that only his corrections to the works of Guglielmo Grataroli, the Protestant physician from Bergamo, were ever formally adopted. Rossi's expurgations make up about three-quarters of Grataroli's entry in the 1607 *Index expurgatorius*, but even though they appear verbatim in print, Rossi's manuscript suggestions included still more expurgations that were either ignored or deemed unnecessary by censors in Rome, in particular his attention to matters concerning physiognomy.[43] Despite his prolific participation in censorship efforts, Rossi's contribution to the long-term integration of Protestant knowledge in Catholic Italy was extremely limited. Catholic authorities called on physicians like Rossi to lend

---

43   Baldini and Spruit, *Catholic Church and Modern Science*, vol.1, t. 2, 1887, 1889-1893.

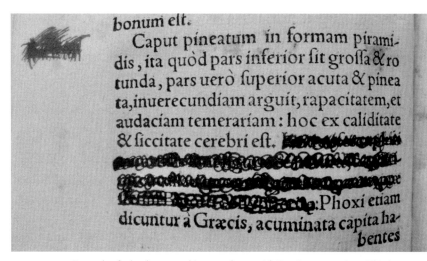

FIGURE 1   *Example of a book censored in accordance with Rossi's expurgations. This is a*
section on physiognomy that mocks the clergy, from Guglielmo Grataroli's Opuscula
(Basel, 1554). The expurgated passage reads: "Many of the Genovese have this form
and nature, and many are hooded – those they call religious are particularly
cowards and hypocrites" ("Ianuenses ut plurimum talis sunt figurae & naturae, &
plurimi cucullati quos religiosos vocant, praesertim Bigotti & hypocrite"). Rossi was
concerned that this passage was damaging to the reputation of the clergy. This copy
is held in the National Library of Medicine in Washington, DC, NLM ID: 101083910.

their expertise to expurgation projects, but ultimately the authority for these
decisions lay with ecclesiastics in Rome.

The Mind of the Censor

Since Girolamo Rossi and his family had strong ties to the Catholic Church, we
should perhaps not be surprised that the Vicar Fabio Tempestivo described
Rossi as "a man no less full of zeal and Christian piety than of learning."[44] But
was piety alone enough to induce a learned physician to become a censor?
Perhaps not, but Rossi's biography and personal papers offer glimpses into the
mind of this physician-censor and shed light on Rossi's motivations for expurgating books and the results of these expurgations on how he saw the world.

---

44   ACDF, Index III, vol. VI, f. 5r. Dated 29 February 1601: "Signor Gerollamo Rossi huomo non
       meno ricco di zelo et pietà Christiana che di scienze."

Girolamo Rossi's uncle, Giovan Battista Rossi, for whom he was a secretary as a young man, was an important and high profile reformer in the post-Tridentine period.[45] Giovan Battista Rossi is remembered fondly in the *Foundations* of Saint Teresa of Avila as the head of the Carmelite order who allowed her to continue founding monasteries.[46] Giovan Battista was also one of three monks assigned to correcting the translation of the Catholic Vulgate Bible in 1568.[47] He was rigid in his applications of the rules of Trent and strictly valued obedience and hierarchy within the Church. Some of the rigor of Girolamo Rossi's Catholic piety likely came from his long stays as a young man at his uncle's convent of San Martino ai Monti in Rome. At the very least, we know for certain that Girolamo Rossi's uncle, Giovan Battista, was a respected and admired figure in his nephew the physician's life. Although Giovan Battista died in 1578, he lived on for Girolamo Rossi as an important character in his *History of Ravenna* and as the namesake of his first-born son.[48]

Unlike his uncle or the physician from Imola, Giovan Battista Codronchi, Rossi never took up orders. Instead, he lived his whole life as a lay member of society. He was the father of ten children, and was especially closely involved in the lives of his twin sons, Francesco and Gerardo, who studied law in Padua and graduated in 1599.[49] His correspondence is also full of references and salutations to his wife, Laura, to whom Rossi was married for 37 years and whom he described following her death in 1604 as "a woman with great genius in the administration of domestic matters, but greater still in devotion to God."[50]

Girolamo Rossi is a rather unique figure in the history of medicine, science, and censorship, since he is among the few lay censors who produced a large number of expurgations in the period between 1596 and 1607. For someone like Rossi, the Catholic Church's call for the expertise of lay practitioners gave a family man who was never ordained the chance to participate actively in shaping the Counter-Reformation Church. What his uncle Giovan Battista had

---

45   The most recent study of Giovan Battista Rossi is *Giovanni Battista Rossi: Carmelitano ravennate: Atti del convegno organizzato a Ravenna il 14/15 dicembre 1979* (Ravenna, 1980).

46   Giovan Battista Rossi's visit to Avila and his meetings with Teresa are the subject of chapter 2 of the *Book of the Foundations of Saint Teresa*.

47   The others were Giovani Morone, Marcantonio Arnulio, and Giuglielmo Sirleto. This is mentioned in, for example, Francesco Saverio de Feller, *Dizionario storico ossia storia compendiata* (Venice, 1834), vol. IX, 298.

48   Giovan Battista Rossi makes several appearances in Girolamo Rossi's *History of Ravenna*, see Rossi, *Storie Ravennati*, 8, 754-755, 758.

49   For a list of his children see BCRa, Mob. 3. 1 B, n. 5, f. 507r.

50   Ginanni, *Memorie*, 315: "magno in rei domesticae administratione ingenio, sed maiori in Deum pietate."

done as monk by volunteering his expertise in philology and languages to correct the Vulgate Bible, Girolamo did in the field of medicine by expurgating the works of Protestants in order to make available and render orthodox the most useful medical learning of a confessionalized world.

Rossi's efforts to correct medical books did not stop with those written by Protestants that he expurgated as part of a local congregation of censors. Building on his own previous work correcting the pirated edition of his *On Distillation*, Rossi once again took up his pen this time to correct and censor his own work. In an undated draft of a document titled *Disputation of Girolamo Rossi on the Quantity of those Qualities which are Attributed to Elements*, Rossi removed his own references to prohibited authors.[51] In a passage describing the errors of Aristotle for which Girolamo Cardano's works served as an important corrective, Rossi praised Cardano as "a man most learned anywhere and of greatest ingenuity" (see Fig. 2). Rossi clearly felt that this praise was perhaps too unqualified to be applied to someone like Cardano, who had been tried several times by the Inquisition and whose name appeared on the Index of Prohibited Books. Rossi excised the praise of his intellect and learning with a thin line of ink.[52] Throughout the treatise Rossi continued to edit his text and censor his remarks pertaining to Cardano, removing his praise of Cardano's great learning [*doctrina*] and his eloquent writing.[53]

Rossi, acting as censor, reader, and author all at once, also removed some of his praise of Ortensio Lando, the author of the *Paradoxes* and translator of Luther's works and More's *Utopia* into Italian (and also a student of medicine).[54] Rossi had originally praised Lando as a man of "extraordinary power of speaking, of the greatest festivity and charm in addition."[55] His censored version removed this high praise, leaving only the author's name and inserting the title of his book, the *Paradoxes*.[56] Rossi also edited Giovanni Battista da Monte's

51   "De earum q[uae] elementis tribuuntur qualitatum, quantitate, Hieronymi Rubei Ravennatis Disputatio," BCRa, Mob. 3. 1 B, n. 4, ff. 405r-414v.

52   Ibid., f. 405r.

53   Ibid., ff. 406r, 408v.

54   Paul Grendler, *Critics of the Italian World, 1530-1560: Anton Francesco Doni, Nicolò Franco & Ortensio Lando* (Madison, WI, 1969), 22. On Lando generally, see Simonetta Adorni Braccesi and Simone Ragagli, "Lando, Ortensio," *DBI*, vol. 63, 451-459.

55   BCRa, Mob. 3. 1 B, n. 4, f. 410r. The Latin reads, "Hortensius Landus, vi dicendi egregia, summa festivitate, et venustate coniuncta, suis paradoxa." There has been a renewed interest in Lando's work in recent years. For his *Paradossi*, see Ortensio Lando, *Paradossi: Cioè sentenze fuori del comun parere*, ed. Antonio Corsaro (Rome, 2000); and Patrizia Grimaldi Pizzorno, *The Ways of Paradox from Lando to Donne* (Florence, 2007).

56   BCRa, Mob. 3. 1 B, n. 4, f. 410r.

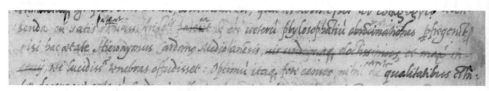

FIGURE 2   *Girolamo Rossi censored his praise of Girolamo Cardano in one of his own manu-*
scripts. The passage above, that Rossi expurgated read, "Girolamo Cardano of Milan,
a man most learned anywhere and of greatest ingenuity" ("Hieronymus Cardanus
Mediolanensis, vir undequaque doctissimus, et maxi[mi] ingenii"). COURTESY OF
THE BIBLIOTECA CLASSENSE, RAVENNA, ITALY. BCRA, MOB. 3. 1 B, N. 4, F. 405R.

name from his treatise replacing it with the general and inoffensive "Hic."[57] Although Da Monte's works were never prohibited on the Index, he was renowned among northern Europeans like Theodor Zwinger, and his works were
published posthumously, many by Protestants including Johann Crato von
Krafftheim, Girolamo Donzellini, and Valentinus Lublinus.[58] Either Rossi suspected Da Monte and his texts of guilt by association, or the acts of censoring
and editing a text had become one and the same project for him.

The explicit evidence of self-censorship found in Girolamo Rossi's treatise is
an example of a phenomenon that was likely widespread but rarely left a paper
trail.[59] Traces of self-censorship most often exist through intermediaries, such
as printers seeking imprimaturs or the Italian translator of Jean Bodin's *Démonomanie* (first translated into Italian in 1587), who censored his translation
so that Bodin's work would be permitted.[60] Rossi's edits provide an opportu-

---

57   Ibid., f. 412r.

58   Maria Muccillo, "Da Monte, Giovanni Battista, dettò Montano," *DBI*, vol. 32, 365-367. This
       entry is quite short. For more on Giovan Battista da Monte see Daniela Mugnai Carrara,
       "Le epistole prefatorie sull'ordine dei libri di Galeno di Giovan Battista da Monte: Esigenze
       di metodo e dilemmi editoriali," in Vicenzo Fera and Agostino Guida, eds., *Vetustatis inda-
       gatur: Scritti offerti a Filippo di Benedetto* (Messina, 1999), 207-234; Silvia Ferretto, *Maestri
       per il metodo di trattar le cose: Bassiano Lando, Giovan Battista da Monte e la scienza della
       medicina nel XVI secolo* (Padua, 2012); and Nancy G. Siraisi, *Avicenna in Renaissance Italy:
       The* Canon *and medical teaching in Italian Universities after 1500* (Princeton, NJ, 1987), 194-
       202.

59   On the ambitious (and perhaps impossible) interpretation of early modern works in light
       of self-censorship, see Annabel Patterson, *Censorship and Interpretation: The Conditions of
       Writing and Reading in Early Modern England* (Madison, WI, 1984).

60   Michaela Valente, *Bodin in Italia: La* Démonomanie des sorciers *e le vincende della sua
       traduzione* (Florence, 1999), 75-146. For other studies dealing with literary self-censorship
       see: Ugo Rozzo, "Gli 'Hecatommithi' all'Indice," *La Bibliofilia,* 92 (1991), 21-51; and Luigi

nity to reconstruct the kinds of things that might have been said, even by pious, orthodox Catholics, in an unrestricted intellectual climate.

We might also imagine the pain or dissonance that Rossi felt, as he expurgated his own works alongside those written by esteemed, though unorthodox, colleagues. It seems significant that, with the exception of the works by Thomas Erastus, all of the books that Rossi censored were not only part of Italian culture, but mostly written by Rossi's fellow Italians, and all of these authors spent time living on the peninsula or studying in Italian universities. Several of the physicians whose works Rossi would later expurgate, he praised glowingly in the first edition of his own *On Distillation,* though in the index the entries for Conrad Gesner, Hieronymus Brunschwig, Girolamo Cardano, Jean de Roquetaillade, Oribasius, Philipp Ulstad, and Ramon Llull qualified each of these authors as "lapsus."[61] It is no wonder that taking up his pen to censor his colleagues also led Rossi to look back critically at his own work. As Ugo Rozzo has eloquently written of the changing status of book collections, we have seen the "theological and cultural contradictions in which even sincere Catholic intellectuals found themselves, who from one day to the next saw their precious libraries transformed into 'prohibited libraries.'"[62] Living amidst this culture of censorship forced an unstable relationship between Catholic physicians and the works of not only their most celebrated colleagues, but even their own writings.

Conclusion

Girolamo Rossi was a pious physician who embraced the task of expurgation and integrated the Tridentine goals of individual, social, and intellectual reform into his career as a medical professional.[63] In his global, comparative study of censorship, Robert Darnton points out that coercion alone cannot

---

     Firpo, "Correzioni d'autore coatte," in *Studi e problemi di critica testuale* (Bologna, 1961), 143-157.

61   Girolamo Rossi, *De distillatione* (Ravenna,1582), ††v, ††2r-v, [††3]r. See the following examples and pages, though of course many of these authors appear repeatedly throughout the text: Thomas Erastus, 125; Arnald of Villanova, 124; Girolamo Cardano, 127.

62   Ugo Rozzo, *Biblioteche italiane del Cinquecento tra Riforma e Controriforma* (Udine, 1994), 28.

63   Ugo Rozzo has posited that beginning in the 1560s, the expurgation of literary texts was "defined and implemented with the uncoerced complicity of the many intellectuals who turned themselves into expurgators." While I agree that Rossi's participation was "uncoerced," it took place in a context of official expurgatory assignments around Italy. See Ugo

sustain systems of control and concludes, "All systems need true believers."[64] Girolamo Rossi was a true believer, even in more senses than Darnton's study imagined, since early modern Catholic censorship inextricably merged the realms of bureaucracy, scholarship, professional expertise, and faith. There were other prolific censors of scientific books like Ambrogio Biturno and Alfonso Chacón, but both of these men were monks, while Rossi presents an unusual case of an active, lay censor whose professional vocation was practicing medicine. Through Rossi's efforts we can gain some intuition into how pious lay professionals responded to the expurgatory moment. The *honorata impresa* was an unwelcome burden to most scholars, yet Rossi seized upon it as an opportunity to engage as a physician in defining the important, orthodox knowledge of Counter-Reformation Catholicism.

Rossi's rich archival trail also allows us to reframe the outcomes of expurgation in terms of readers rather than texts. Rossi's work as a censor changed the way that he read and worked as a physician; when revisiting his own manuscripts, he did so with a pen in hand in order to correct, revise, and ultimately expurgate.[65] Catholic physicians knew that when they read books by certain authors they were obligated to circumscribe their interpretations of those texts. Similarly, when physicians like Rossi published books that they wanted to be read in Italy, they understood that they now needed to read and write more cautiously. While the Index of Prohibited Books was ineffective at producing medical texts that were purely Catholic, cleansed of their references to Protestant authors and theologies, the process of lay expurgation succeeded in training physicians and other professionals to actively censor themselves.

If the culture of censorship created readers who thought like expurgators, this must have been in part because of the long-standing humanist tradition of reading for commonplacing.[66] The humanistically trained Renaissance reader

---

Rozzo, "Italian Literature on the Index," in Fragnito, ed., *Church, Censorship, and Culture,* 194-222, at 222.

64   Darnton, *Censors at Work,* 234.

65   On humanist reading with pen in hand, see Lisa Jardine and Anthony Grafton, "'Studied for Action': How Gabriel Harvey Read His Livy," *Past & Present,* 129 (1990), 30-78. The humanist culture of correction entered into print shops through the role of correctors. This same humanist ethos to purify and correct texts also entered into censorship efforts through the process of expurgation, especially in 1590s and early 1600s. See also Anthony Grafton, *The Culture of Correction in Renaissance Europe* (London, 2011).

66   For an introduction to the vast literature on early modern commonplacing, see Ann Moss, *Printed Commonplace-Books and the Structuring of Renaissance Thought* (Oxford, 1996); Ann Blair, *Too Much to Know,* 62-116; Ann Blair, "Humanist Methods in Natural Philosophy: The Commonplace Book," *Journal of the History of Ideas,* 53 (1992), 541-551.

read with a pen in hand, not to censor, as Girolamo Rossi did, but to mark passages or copy them into commonplace books, like Seneca's industrious bees. It is a short step, then, to arrive at expurgation as the "dark side of commonplacing," marking passages ultimately for removal instead of preservation.[67] During the expurgatory moment, the Catholic Church turned traditional humanist techniques for extracting from books into a new, pious form of reading.

Expurgation was the dark side of commonplacing, and the *Index expurgatorius* of 1607 became something of an anti-commonplace book, delineating what Catholics should not repeat. The *Index expurgatorius* lists fifty authors and the pages in the volume where readers could find the expurgations of their works. Next follows a recapitulation of the rules of the Clementine Index and the kinds of words, images, and ideas that needed to be removed from books in order to read them. Last follow the specifics, organized by author, title, and edition. From Amatus Lusitanus's *Curationum medicinalium*, the Lyon edition of 1580, in *curatione* 9, page 99, readers were instructed to delete text after the words "*ante sua obitum multum vigilaverat*" and up to the phrase "*si qua vero noctes pars, etc.*"[68] The offensive parts of the expurgated passage are obscured through the instructions, and the only full passages that are reproduced are those in which the text sets out to denote how a passage should read after a section has been removed. As a commonplace book, this *Index expurgatorius* was a compilation of readings to be, if not forgotten, then certainly not reused and repurposed by Catholic scholars.[69]

Girolamo Rossi died in Ravenna in 1607, the same year that the *Index expurgatorius* was published.[70] The work by physicians and other lay censors across Italy led to few of the expurgations published within it, but this reference book of prohibited passages to be extracted from important texts laid the groundwork for how licensed readers across the seventeenth century would encounter prohibited books. Ultimately, participating in expurgation taught medical scholars to read like censors, and the eventual publication of the *Index expurgatorius* served as a critical stepping stone toward reintegrating prohibited medical books into Italian collections and libraries.

---

67   I am grateful to Simon Reader for this wonderful turn of phrase.

68   *Indicis librorum expurgandorum in studiosorum gratiam confecti...* (Rome, 1607), 12-13. The missing words removed from between these two indicators are "quia solicitus admodum erat circa divinas preces, quas Hebraei illis diebus noctu effundere ad Deum solent."

69   On willful ignorance and the art of forgetting, see Robert Proctor and Londa Schiebinger, eds., *Agnotology: The Making and Unmaking of Ignorance* (Stanford, CA, 2008).

70   On the complications of publishing the 1607 *Index expurgatorius*, see Gigliola Fragnito, "Un archivio conteso: Le 'carte' dell'Indice tra Congregazione e Maestro del Sacro Palazzo," *Rivista storica italiana*, 119 (2007), 1275-1318.

The Heart of Heresy: Inquisition, Medicine, and False Sanctity

Bradford A. Bouley
University of California Santa Barbara
bouley@ucsb.edu

Abstract

This paper examines the engagement of various officials and tribunals of the Roman Inquisition with the new anatomical studies of the early modern period. It argues that although inquisition officers were frequently very aware of the latest medical theories, they actively chose not to employ anatomical or medical evidence when evaluating the unusual physical symptoms that might be associated with false or affected sanctity. This attitude stands in contrast to the employment of anatomical knowledge by other ecclesiastical institutions – e.g. the Congregation of Rites – and suggests that the Inquisition held a different, and perhaps more modern, view about the relationship between natural knowledge and religion.

Keywords

anatomy – saint – body – inquisition – heart – Rome – Paolo Zacchia

In 1653 Agapito Ugoni, the inquisitor assigned to the city of Vicenza, near Venice, sent two woodcut impressions to the central office of the Roman Inquisition (see Figs. 1, 2).[1] These images portrayed the heart of the medieval

---

* Department of History, Humanities and Social Sciences Building, University of California, Santa Barbara, CA 93106, USA.

1 Ugoni was a native of Brescia, and he served as the Roman Inquisition's appointee in Vicenza from 1652 to 1663. For more information on him, see Anne Jacobson Schutte, *Aspiring Saints: Pretense of Holiness, Inquisition and Gender in the Republic of Venice, 1618-1750* (Baltimore, MD, 2001), 31-34.

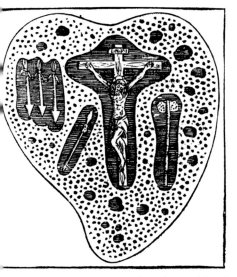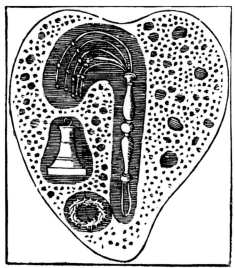

FIGURES 1 AND 2   *Clare of Montefalco's heart. Battista Piergilii da Bevagna, Vita, pp. 14-15 of*
unpaginated front matter. The same images appear in ACDF, St. St. MS
B-4-F, fasc. 11, ff. 3r, 4r.

Augustinian nun, Clare of Montefalco (1268-1308), as her sister nuns reported
they had found it when they dissected her corpse in 1308. In life, Clare had
frequently claimed that Jesus dwelt in her heart. In 1308, her (apparently) liter-
al-minded holy sisters opened her body to investigate the veracity of this asser-
tion. During the autopsy, the nuns discovered wondrous objects within Clare's
heart – a tiny cross, a lance, a crown of thorns, and other instruments of the
passion. Searching further, they found that her gall bladder housed three
stones that were taken to represent the trinity. The nuns and their supporters
believed the instruments of the passion and the stones were proof of Clare's
sanctity.[2] These assertions were hotly contested, and during an attempt to can-
onize Clare begun ten years later, in 1318, a local Franciscan claimed that the

---

2   Enrico Menestò, ed., *Il processo di canonizzazione di Chiara da Montefalco* (Perugia, 1984),
     339-341. For a discussion of Clare's original dissection and its meaning in the context of the
     fourteenth century see Katharine Park, "The Criminal and the Saintly Body: Autopsy and
     Dissection in Renaissance Italy," *Renaissance Quarterly*, 47, (1994), 1-33; eadem, "Relics of a
     Fertile Heart: the 'Autopsy' of Clare of Montefalco," in Anne L. McClanan and Karen Rosoff
     Encarnación, eds., *The Material Culture of Sex, Procreation, and Marriage in Premodern Europe*
     (New York, NY, 2002), 115-133; eadem, *Secrets of Women: Gender, Generation, and the Origins of
     Human Dissection* (New York, NY, 2006).

nuns had, in fact, planted the items.[3] This medieval phase of Clare's canonization ended inconclusively.[4]

Nevertheless, Clare's cult endured and even grew in popularity following the Reformation.[5] In the 1650s a publisher from the same region where Clare had lived began circulating printed *vitae* that included the woodcut impressions as anatomical images of Clare's heart.[6] It was these images that troubled the inquisitor Ugoni. He stated his belief in a letter to the central tribunal of the Roman Inquisition that the images portrayed by the woodcuts "were not authentic." Ugoni, like the medieval Franciscan friar before him, was skeptical of the physical evidence as a record of Clare's sanctity. Given his concerns, Ugoni suspended the license to print the *vita*. He then sought approval for this action from the Holy Office in Rome.[7]

Although Ugoni's concerns in 1653 might seem similar to those of the fourteenth century, the context was strikingly different. In large measure this was owing to the fact that, during the intervening three hundred years, the prestige of medicine in general, and anatomy in particular, had risen greatly. A vigorous revival of Galen had occurred, numerous master works of anatomy had been produced, and empirical methods had been introduced as a key to making knowledge of the human body.[8] The Catholic Church had also undergone profound change that deeply affected its stance towards medicine. Given these

---

3 Menestò, ed., *Il processo,* 435. "Unde habeo violentam suspicionem quod, sicut dicitur, illa signa cordis eius fuerunt facta artificiose ab una sorore de Fulgineo, que reclusa morabatur in monasterio nominato, que cum manibus suis subtiliter operabatur, que fuit mortua modico tempore interiecto."

4 Park, "Relics of a Fertile Heart," 121; André Vauchez, *Sainthood in the Later Middle Ages,* trans. Jean Birrell (New York, NY, 1997), 523. Vauchez notes that Clare's canonization was the first to include a systematic and skeptical inquiry into the miracles of the saint. Clare was eventually canonized in 1881.

5 Roberto Tollo, ed., *Santa Chiara da Montefalco: Culto, storia e arte* (Tolentino, 2009). Her cult was popular enough in the early seventeenth century for Pope Clement VIII (d. 1605) to cite it as one that concerned him when he sought to overhaul canonization procedures. See Biblioteca Apostolica Vaticana (BAV), MS Barberini Latini (Barb. Lat.) 2810, 341.

6 Battista Piergilii da Bevagna, *Vita della B. Chiara della croce da Montefalco* (Foligno, 1640), [14-15] (unpaginated front matter).

7 Archivio della Congregazione per la Dottrina della Fede (ACDF), Stanza Storica (St. St.) MS B-4-F, fasc. 11, f. 5r. "Lo supplico avisarmi, se l'impressione del core della B. Chiara da' Montefalco mon[ac]a Agostiniana da' Montefalco, di cui mando un'essemplare, sia lecita, havendome io sospeso la licenza, per non sapere, se sia cosa autentica [...][.] Humiliss[im] o Ded[i]c[issi]mo et Obblig[atissi]mo serv[itor]e F. Agapito Ugoni Inq[uisto]re."

8 For surveys of the changes taking place in medicine in the sixteenth and seventeenth centuries see Mary Lindemann, *Medicine and Society in Early Modern Europe* (New York,

innovations, it had become common for ecclesiastical institutions to seek out medical or anatomical advice when judging the merits of a saint, a dubious miracle, or some other phenomenon which might involve the human body.[9]

Despite this new prestige of medicine and the cooperation between theologians and medical experts, the Roman Inquisition was suspicious of physical evidence as an indicator of sanctity. Ugoni's skepticism of Clare's case was merely emblematic of the attitude in general, and his actions received approval from the central branch of the Roman Inquisition.[10] Such caution over medical testimony occurred notwithstanding the fact that members of the Roman Inquisition regularly interacted with medical professionals and frequently held them on retainer.

This paper will explore the reticence of the Roman Inquisition to use medical evidence in spiritual matters, beginning first with a brief survey of the current scholarship on false saints and the role of medicine in evaluating them, before turning to the early modern consensus that medicine and theology were complementary fields when it came to understanding the holy. A survey of specific cases in which bodily evidence featured prominently in trials before the Roman Inquisition will demonstrate that inquisitors hesitated to use medical expertise in such cases not due to suspicion against natural philosophy or current medical knowledge on the part of Roman inquisitors. Rather, the Roman Inquisition's failure to employ medical professionals for discernment of sanctity most likely stems from three contributing factors: the potentially prohibitive cost of employing medical experts, the notoriety that such involvement might bring to dubious cases, and the fact that, by the time a case for pretense of sanctity had reached the offices of the Inquisition, the physical

NY, 2010); Roy Porter, "Medical Science," in Roy Porter, ed., *The Cambridge History of Medicine* (New York, NY, 2006), 136-175.

9   Bradford Bouley, *Pious Postmortems: Anatomy, Sanctity, and the Catholic Church in Early Modern Europe* (Philadelphia, PA, 2017); Jacalyn Duffin, *Medical Miracles: Doctors, Saints, and Healing in the Modern World* (New York, NY, 2009); David Gentilcore, *Healers and Healing in Early Modern Italy* (New York, NY, 1998), 187-198; Fernando Vidal, "Miracles, Science, and Testimony in Post-Tridentine Saint-Making," *Science in Context*, 20 (2007), 481-508.

10   ACDF, MS Decreta Sancti Officii 1653, f. 104v. Although the *decreta* states that the matter was considered, there does not seem to have been a ruling issued either to confirm or deny Ugoni's action, which means that the ban would have remained in effect in the Veneto. For a recent discussion of the interaction between the central tribunal of the Roman Inquisition and its peripheral offices, see Thomas F. Mayer, *The Roman Inquisition on the Stage of Italy, c. 1590-1640* (Philadelphia, PA, 2014).

evidence was usually considered too dubious to merit actual medical consideration.

Scholarship on Medicine and False Sanctity

In recent years there have been numerous studies on the phenomenon of false or affected sanctity.[11] The term 'affected sanctity' was a contemporary one used to describe a person who was considered to be counterfeiting signs of holiness or perhaps, even worse, was endowed with saint-like abilities by Satan so as to lead the faithful astray. Although the concept had existed since the early years of the Church, it had only begun to be regularly prosecuted by the Roman Inquisition in the early seventeenth century, with the Spanish Inquisition having become aware of this pretense and taking action against malingerers slightly earlier.[12] Historians consider this change in attitude and beginning of prosecutions to have stemmed from the attempt within the Catholic Church to rearticulate the meaning of holiness in the same period.[13] It was, after all, just at this moment that Church officials began to elevate a number of people to sainthood after a long pause following the Reformation. The election of five saints in 1622 was a key moment in the unfolding of a newly defined sanctity.[14]

---

11   Elena Brambilla, *Corpi invasi e viaggi dell'anima: Santità, possessione, esorcismo dalla teologia barocca alla medicina illuminista* (Rome, 2010); Andrew Keitt, *Inventing the Sacred: Imposture, Inquisition and the Boundaries of the Supernatural in Golden Age Spain* (Boston, MA, 2005); Schutte, *Aspiring Saints;* eadem, "Pretense of Holiness in Italy Investigations and Persecutions (1581-1876)," *Rivista di storia e letteratura religiosa,* 27 (2001), 299-321; Moshe Sluhovsky, *Believe not Every Spirit: Possession, Mysticism and Discernment in Early Modern Catholicism* (Chicago, IL, 2007); Gabriella Zarri, ed., *Finzione e santità tra medioevo ed età moderna* (Turin, 1991). The literature on false sanctity is vast and growing. These citations represent merely a sample from the relevant literature.

12   Schutte, *Aspiring Saints,* 42; Giuseppe Dalla Torre, "Santità ed economia processuale: L'esperienza giuridica da Urbano VIII e Benedetto XIV," in *Finzione e santità,* 231-263; Gabriella Zarri, "'Vera' santità, 'simulata' santità: Ipotesi e riscontri," in Zarri, ed., *Finzione e santità,* 9-36.

13   Schutte, *Aspiring Saints,* 73; Zarri, "'Vera' santità," 11.

14   On the rearticulation of sanctity following the Reformation, see Peter Burke, "How to be a Counter Reformation Saint," in Kaspar von Greyerz, ed., *Religion and Society in Early Modern Europe 1500-1800* (London, 1984), 45-55; Simon Ditchfield, "How not to Be a Counter-Reformation Saint: The Attempted Canonization of Pope Gregory X, 1622-45," *Papers of the British School at Rome,* 60 (1992), 379-422; idem, "Tridentine Worship and the Cult of the Saints," in R. Po-Chia Hsia, ed., *The Cambridge History of Christianity,* vol. 6 (New York, NY, 2007), 201-224; Miguel Gotor, *Chiesa e santità nell'Italia moderna* (Rome, 2004); idem,

Although everyone seemed to agree that false saints were a real problem, it was difficult in practice to separate those truly touched by God – or the Devil – from the impostors. The efforts to 'discern spirits' became a major preoccupation in early modern Europe, and historian Stephen Haliczer has even called the attempt to demonstrate connections between man and the divine "the dominant intellectual concern in sixteenth- and seventeenth-century Europe."[15] That is, understanding the workings of God in this world during a period of profound religious crisis was a central preoccupation for a great number of people across all confessional divides. Unusual events – such as wonder-working individuals – were thought to be ways to read God's movements on Earth.[16] For this reason, many organizations, including the Tribunal of the Rota in Rome and the Congregation of Rites, both from within the Church, turned to medicine as the field that could best help identify true sanctity. As experts on the body, physicians were ideally trained to determine whether or not signs of sanctity such as the stigmata, incredibly long fasts, and other miracles were due to some natural but obscure phenomenon, Satan, or God himself.[17] Physicians, as we shall see below, even touted their ability to act as discerners of spirits.

Nevertheless, despite the employment of physicians to discern spirits by other tribunals within the Church, the Roman Inquisition does not appear to have employed any sort of medical professionals in this way. Historian Anne Schutte attributes this failure to use medical evidence to

> tunnel vision: inquisitors simply had not bothered to acquaint themselves with parallel and potentially complementary developments in medicine. As learned and widely read as they were, their mental universe did not extend beyond their own disciplines of theology and canon law.[18]

I beati del Papa: Santità, inquisizione e obbedienza in età moderna (Florence, 2002); Giovanni Papa, *Le cause di canonizzazione nel primo periodo della congregazione dei Riti (1588-1634)* (Rome, 2001).

15 Stephen Haliczer, *Between Exaltation and Infamy: Female Mystics in the Golden Age of Spain* (New York, NY, 2002), 11.

16 Stuart Clark, *Thinking with Demons: The Idea of Witchcraft in Early Modern Europe* (New York, NY, 1997), 151-281; Lorraine Daston and Katharine Park, *Wonders and the Order of Nature, 1150-1750* (New York, NY, 1998), 215-254; Moshe Sluhovsky, *Believe not Every Spirit*, 1-12; Keitt, *Inventing the Sacred*, 235.

17 Keitt, *Inventing the Sacred*, 155-156.

18 Schutte, *Aspiring Saints*, 147.

This does not always seem to have been the case, though, since many of the individuals who served the Roman Inquisition also worked for either the Congregation of Rites or the Tribunal of the Rota.[19] These two organizations began, especially after 1600, to use medical expertise routinely to determine whether something outside the boundaries of nature – whether demonic or divine – had occurred.[20] Inquisitors must have decided, therefore, not to use medical expertise as one of the ways in which they assessed claims of extraordinary human holiness.

That the Roman Inquisition did not rely on expert medical knowledge for the discernment of spirits suggests not just a difference of opinion between this and other early modern ecclesiastical institutions, but a different view on how nature operated. The prevailing medical and theological view up until the middle of the seventeenth century had been that body and spirit were intimately connected. Therefore, changes in one would manifest in the other.[21] But in relying only on theological expertise to evaluate potential holiness the Inquisition implied that physical evidence did not matter in such cases. That is, spirit and body were different entities. Although this was certainly not their overt intention in doing so, the Inquisition's activities in some ways endorsed a new way of looking at the relationship between body and spirit. That their attitude was a departure from the norm becomes even more apparent when viewed against the background of medical, theological, and legal consensus that had been established by the early seventeenth century, that medicine was a central part of the discernment of spirits.

Calls for Collaboration

The Roman Inquisition's failure to deploy physical evidence in the discernment of spirits presents a contrast to how contemporaries felt sanctity – or a lack thereof – should be evaluated. The consensus in the sixteenth and seventeenth centuries was that the body was the key to understanding the true spirit of an individual. Indeed, theologians and canon lawyers associated with the

---

19   Peter Godman, *The Saint as Censor Robert Bellarmine Between Inquisition and Index* (Boston, MA, 2000), 91-92. Godman has noted here that some inquisitors also worked for the Rota as well and were involved with saint making. Francisco Peña, for example, was deacon of the Rota and yet also consulted for the Roman Inquisition.

20   Bouley, *Pious Postmortems*.

21   For a brief discussion of the medical and theological concepts behind this in the early seventeenth century, see Brambilla, *Corpi invasi*, 66-74.

Congregation of Rites – that is, the branch of the Church charged with evaluating the cases of prospective saints – regularly relied on anatomical evidence, interpreted by expert physicians, as part of their judgment of sanctity.[22] Likewise, Protestants also believed that holiness could be visible in the body of the deceased. Theodore Beza (1519-1605), Calvin's successor in Geneva, drawing from the cases of several Protestant martyrs, concluded that the failure of corpses to rot despite being long dead was a sign of their holiness. There was similarly widespread debate over whether or not Martin Luther could have died of a stroke, since such sudden death was not thought to be not characteristic of a holy man.[23] Holiness was therefore believed both by Protestants and Catholics to be visible in the body.[24]

Similarly, theologians across the confessional divide believed that signs of immorality would also leave their mark on the body. The French Protestant martyrologist Jean Crespin (1520-1572) recounted in one work the various ways in which especially evil people's bodies might be prone to disease and disability, which he took as signs of their depravity manifested physically.[25] According to both Catholic and Protestant authors, the bodies of various popes became wracked by maladies as an indication of their impious lives.[26] Catholic polemicists attributed numerous bodily ailments to Protestant reformers. The Jesuit Théophile Raynaud (1583-1663), for example, described how Martin Luther's body rotted rapidly after death, despite multiple efforts to embalm it. In Raynaud's recounting, such rot was a clear mark of Luther's unholy life.[27] The Catholic author Johannes Cochlaeus (1479-1552) attributed a strange heart palpitation to Luther as a sign that the devil had taken over that organ, and hence, his body and mind.[28] Jerome Bolsec (d. 1584), a Carmelite monk and medical dabbler, published a hostile biography of John Calvin in which he asserted that

22   Bouley, *Pious Postmortems*, 39-70.

23   Hartmann Grisar, *Luther*, trans. E.M. Lamond, vol. 4 (St. Louis, MO, 1917), 380. On concerns about sudden death more generally see Maria Pia Donato, *Sudden Death: Medicine and Religion in Eighteenth-Century Rome* (Farnham, 2014).

24   On the medieval background to this belief, see Park, "The Criminal and the Saintly Body."

25   Parker, "Diseased Bodies," 1266.

26   Bradford Bouley, "Papal Anatomy in the News: Bodies and Politics in the Early Modern Catholic World," *Sixteenth Century Journal* (forthcoming).

27   Theophilis Raynaudus, *De incorruptione cadaverum, occasione de mortui foeminei corporis post aliquot secula incorrupti, nuper refossi Carpentoracti* (Avignon, 1665), 193: "Sed et Lutheri cadaver quantumvis summa cura conditum, etiam priusquam sepulchro inferretur foetorem emisisse qui ferri non poterat."

28   Johannes Cochlaeus, "The Deeds and Writings of Dr. Martin Luther from the Year of the Lord 1517 to the year 1546," in Elizabeth Vandiver, Ralph Keen, and Thomas D. Franzel, eds.

the latter died of syphilis, a disease with obvious negative connotations.[29] In short, there was widespread consensus that especially holy or evil individuals would show signs of their spiritual state.

Physicians, for their part, held similar convictions and advocated for their role in discerning a person's spiritual state through bodily evidence. In addition to the numerous medical professionals whom the Congregation of Rites employed to evaluate miracles during canonization proceedings, several physicians wrote manuals in which they advertised their skills as evaluating spiritual signs in the human body. The mid-seventeenth-century Roman physician Paolo Zacchia (1584-1659) provided a guide for discerning spirits in his *Medical-Legal Questions*, which was published in ten books beginning with the first volume in 1621 and a first full edition of all books issued in 1651.[30] In particular, he advised medical experts on how to judge whether stigmata, extended fasts, ecstasies, raptures, and even unusual diseases had natural, preternatural, or supernatural causes.[31] These were all potential signs of sanctity, and determining whether they were inspired by God – i.e. supernatural – was a difficult task, which Zacchia and other physicians were only too happy to help canon lawyers evaluate – for a fee.[32] Zacchia also specifically advertised to his readers that he was able to spot one such false female saint who had deceived others, because he knew her "inside and under her skin" and that was how he could be so sure.[33] Such statements suggested to readers that Zacchia's medical and

---

        and trans., *Luther's Lives: Two Contemporary Accounts of Martin Luther,* (New York, NY, 2002), 302-303.

29   John Wilkinson, *The Medical History of the Reformers: Martin Luther, John Calvin, John Knox* (Edinburgh, 2001), 59.

30   Maria Gigliola and Renzo Villata, "Paolo Zacchia, la medicina come sapere globale e la 'sfida' al diritto," in Alessandro Pastore and Giovanni Rossi, eds., *Paolo Zacchia alle origini della medicina legale 1584-1659* (Milan, 2008), 12.

31   Paolo Zacchia, *Quaestionum medico-legalium tomi tres. Editio nova, a variis mendis purgata, passimque interpolata, et novis recentiorum authorum inventis ac observationibus aucta ...* (Frankfurt, 1666), Lib II Tit. I, Quaest. XVIII (on lymphatics, demoniacs, ecstatics, etc.), Lib IV, Tit I, Quaest. VI (on fake ecstasies and raptures), Lib IV, Tit. I, Quaest. VII (on unusually long fasts), Lib VII, Tit. IV, Quaest. I (on stigmata), as well as other sections in book IV on miracles. See also Elena Brambilla, "Patologie miracolose e diaboliche nelle Quaestiones medico-legales di Paolo Zacchia," in *Paolo Zacchia alle origini della medicina legale,* 138-162.

32   On the boundaries of nature, see Daston and Park, *Wonders and the Order of Nature,* 120-128.

33   Zacchia, *Quaestionum medico-legalium* (1666), 254: "Vidi ego mulierem mihi satis notam, quae se, ubi frequens hominum coetus in templis, sacrisque locis convenisset, raptam in Ecstasim effingebat, & admiratione non parva dignum erat, quam apte simularet. Stabat

anatomical knowledge made him a supremely qualified judge of a person's spiritual merits.

Numerous other physicians in the sixteenth and seventeenth centuries similarly attempted to bill themselves as experts in understanding the interaction between the physical and the spiritual. Marcello Donati (1538-1602), a physician from Mantua, seems also to have engaged in some medical discernment of spirits. In particular, he recounted a number of cases in which supposedly miraculous fasts were reinterpreted in the light of medical evidence as being within the range of normal human endurance. He also examined a case of unusual vomiting that seemed to have been demonically inspired. He concluded, instead, that this malady was rooted in a humoral imbalance.[34] Extreme fasting featured regularly in – especially female – saints' lives during this period, whereas unusual vomiting was considered a sign of demonic possession.[35] Thus, Donati interpreted and naturalized both miraculous and sinister bodily abnormalities associated with spiritual problems. In a vein similar to Donati and Zacchia, the Roman physician Angelo Vittori (1547-after 1633) regularly testified for the Tribunal of the Rota – the highest ecclesiastical court – about wondrous bodily abnormalities. Vittori printed a collection of some of his more important results, many of which included evaluations of prospective saints' bodies.[36] These physicians are merely representative of a wider trend, and other collections of case studies advertised various physicians' willingness

---

extensis brachiis in Crucis modum, palpebris immobilibus, oculis fixis, & per horae spatium, ac ultra, eo in actu perseverabat. Interdum veluti ad coelum volatura, & in aerem se elevatura corpus attollebat, illud mirum in modum extendens; sed admirationem omnem superare mihi visum est, quod vultum in mille colores vel ictu oculi commutaret; nam modo rubescebat; & quasi ardore quodam incendi videbatur, modo adeo pallescebat, ut quasi emortua langueret, denuo, ac dicto citius, rubore perfundebatur ac denique veluti animo deficiens ad seipsam redire simulabat, ita ut circumstantes omnes eam divino raptu prehensam pro sancta venerarentur, & ad illius vestimenta devotionis ergo tangenda, mulierculae & homunciones aderant, acurrerent, non sine mei ipsius risu, & multo majori, ut credo, ipsiusmet foemina derisu, quam ego quidem intus & in cute agnoscebam; erat autem Sicula."

34   Marcello Donato, *De medica historia mirabili libri sex* (Mantua, 1586), ff. 194v, 196r-196v.

35   On fasting and female sanctity, see Rudolph M. Bell, *Holy Anorexia* (Chicago, IL, 1987); Caroline Bynum, *Holy Feast and Holy Fast: The Religious Significance of Food to Medieval Women* (Berkeley, CA, 1987). On the connection between vomiting and possession in the early modern period, see Brambilla, *Corpi invasi*, 82-84.

36   Angelo Vittori, *Medicae consultationes* (Rome, 1640), 381-445. In these pages, he testifies about miracles for Ignatius of Loyola, Francis Xavier, and Filippo Neri.

to use their abilities to interpret the connection between bodily wondrousness and the spirit.[37]

In sum, a consensus existed among experts that theology and medicine could cooperate when it came to interpreting possibly miraculous or demonic signs in the human body. Even Inquisition manuals took up this call, and inquisitorial writers, including Eliseo Masini, Francisco Peña, and Giorgio Polacco, advocated a cooperation between medical, legal, and theological expertise when it came to vetting the potentially holy or the possibly demonic.[38] Nevertheless, representatives of the Roman Inquisition almost entirely refrained from using medicine in the discernment of spirits. Several cases will illustrate this reticence and point to its causes.

Some Case Studies

In the 1660s Lucia Gambona, a tertiary of the Ursulines living with her mother in Gentilino, in the Italian diocese of Como, came to the attention of the Roman Inquisition's officers in Milan.[39] Gambona had been experiencing a variety of visions accompanied by unusual physical symptoms that many attributed to the divine, but which some feared had more nefarious origins. In particular, witnesses reported that she had been inflicted with stigmata, including a series of bloody puncture wounds in her head that mirrored Jesus's injury from the crown of thorns.[40] She also was reputed to have a heart which beat strongly, irregularly, and was incredibly hot. This was attributed to Jesus's presence in her heart – a physical ailment similar to that of Clare of Montefalco.[41] Concerned about these symptoms, the Inquisition transferred Gambona to Milan in 1661 so that she could be more closely observed by ecclesiastical

---

37   Paulus Lentulus, *Historia admiranda, de prodigiosa Apolloniae Schreierae, virginis in agro Bernensi, inedia* (Bern, 1604); Fortunio Liceti, *De his qui diu vivunt sine alimento libri quatuor* (Padua, 1612); Pietro Piperno, *De magicis affectibus* (Naples, 1634).

38   Eliseo Masini, *Sacro arsenale: Ovvero pratica dell'Uffizio della Santa Inquisizione* (Rome, 1730), 297-298; Francisco Peña, *Directorium inquisitorum F. Nicolai Eymerici ordinis praed. cum commentariis Francisci Peñae sacrae theologiae ac juris utriusque doctoris* (Rome, 1587), 439, 629; Giorgio Polacco, *Pratiche per discerner lo spirito buono dal maluagio, e per conoscer gl'indemoniati, e maleficiati* (Bologna, 1638), 118-119.

39   Paola Vismara, "Gambona, Lucia," in Adriano Prosperi, ed., *Dizionario storico dell'Inquisizione* (Pisa, 2010), vol. 2, 643.

40   ACDF, St. St. MS C-1-F, fasc. 2, p. 130.

41   ACDF, St. St. MS C-1-F, fasc. 2, p. 108.

and expert medical authorities.[42] Gambona's case, which was reported on in detail from this point forward, typifies how the Inquisition used medicine in such instances. Despite the fact that she was afflicted by a variety of unusual physical and apparently miraculous ailments, physicians were never asked about the origins of her bodily problems. Rather, they were only tasked with helping manage her pain and sickness.

One example of how medical professionals were used in her case comes from more than a decade into her long observation by Inquisition and other officials. While under watchful eyes in Milan, on March 2, 1679, Gambona awoke at midnight with "acute pain" in her head, on the right side "below her breast," and generally, all over her body.[43] These pains clearly mirrored the locations of the stigmata that she had endured in the past – the injury on her right side echoing Jesus's lance wound, and the head representing the crown of thorns. According to the Inquisition's records, Gambona's confessor heard her screams despite being "in his room in the house." He was then concerned enough about Gambona's pain to fetch both the father inquisitor assigned to her case and the *medico di casa* Giovan Battista Mogno.[44] Her confessor "had her show them the place of the pain and he said that he had seen beneath the same breast a red mark as long and as wide as a finger."[45] The inquisitor then asked to see the place where she hurt and was told that the pain had ceased.[46] Meanwhile, the confessor, "to determine whether or not she had a fever," felt her pulse, but could not find it. The *medico*, Mogno, did the same and confirmed that he also could not find a pulse. No further interpretation was given of this ambivalent physical evidence, and after a few more hours of observation the inquisitor departed.[47]

---

42 ACDF, St. St. MS C-1-E, f. 1v. "Di Maggio 1661 fu per questa divotione condotta a Milano in casa del S[ignor] Giulio Cesare Lucini nipote dell'Arciprete ministro del S[ant] Off[iti]o et un oratore per la Città di Como ove anco si trova."

43 ACDF, St. St. MS C-1-F, fasc. 2, p. 267. "Di un hora di notte dice che ci sente nel capo dolori acuti, e nel lato d[i]ritto sotto la mammella, e nel corpo tutto [...] e li dolori dice che li durano tutta la notte."

44 Ibid., pp. 267-268.

45 Ibid., p. 268. "Li fece egli mostrare dalla donna il luogo del Dolore, e disse che vede sotto la medesima mammella un segno ro[sse]ggiante di lun[g]hezza e larghezza come d'un dito."

46 Ibid., p. 268.

47 Ibid.: "Toccagli il pulso per accertarsi di una feb[b]re, ma non trovò nemeno il pulso [...] [.] Il medesimo fece il S[igno]r. Gio[van] Batt[ist]a Mogno Medico di Casa et egli parve trovò la donna priva del pulso."

This scene is rich with evidence that demonstrates the disconnect between the contemporary belief in the intimate connection between the body and the spirit, and the Inquisition's attitude towards bodily signs of sanctity. Gambona's confessor tried to promote her case by demonstrating physical evidence of her holiness. Despite being in another room he was aware of the pains she was experiencing and ran quickly to get both the inquisitor and the house doctor. This suggests that he was actively listening and looking for such evidence, and then called upon the two people who could actually classify it as being a non-natural malady. Otherwise, if he was just concerned about her pain, he would have called on the *medico* and perhaps someone more sympathetic to Gambona's plight than the inquisitor. Then, rather than letting them explore Gambona's ailments for themselves, the confessor guided them through what was happening, indicating how and where they might find signs of her connection with the divine. He even went so far to take her pulse before the medical professional had a chance to examine her. Such eagerness suggests that he was encouraging the use of physical evidence in verifying her case.

Unfortunately, the evidence seems not to have been very compelling, as it apparently disappeared when the inquisitor looked for it. The inquisitor, furthermore, did not instruct the *medico* to try to search for the now hidden ailment, but rather just left when nothing else seemed to be happening.[48] The physical manifestation of Gambona's unusual connection with either the divine or the demonic was unimportant for the inquisitor.

In a similar case from 1659, a Dominican tertiary from Naples, Giovanna Cesarena, was reputed to survive for a long time on only bread and water, and to go into raptures in which her body remained totally insensible to her surroundings.[49] Numerous medical writers, including Paolo Zacchia, provide lengthy discussions of how to medically determine whether such behavior was false, demonically inspired, or a gift from God.[50] Nevertheless, a *medico* appears to have been consulted in this case only to see whether or not Cesarena's health was endangered by the conditions of her house arrest.[51] The unnamed medical practitioner was not asked about the possible origins of Cesarena's unusual somatic signs. In both these cases, the inquisitors could have easily asked a medical expert about the origin of unusual physical symptoms, but chose not to.

---

48 ACDF, St. St. MS C-1-F, fasc. 2, p. 268.

49 ACDF, St. St. MS C-1-G, f. 3r.

50 Zacchia, *Quaestiones medico-legales,* Lib IV, Tit I, Quaest.VI: De ecstasi, & raptu; Lib IV Tit. I, Quaest. VII: De longo iejunio.

51 ACDF, St. St. C-1-G, f. 33r.

One reason why these inquisitors likely did not seek out medical testimony was because Gambona's and Cesarena's physical signs – however unusual or wondrous – could not be counted as being of divine origin because of who these women were. As another inquisition trial, that of Sister Maria Cristina Rovoles of Sicily in 1680, clearly illustrates, low-born women were more likely to have unusual ailments attributed to natural or demonic origins than to divine ones. In the Inquisition process against Rovoles, the recording notary states that numerous witnesses observed red marks on her hands, feet, and left side, which seemed to mirror the stigmata.[52] Even more impressive, though, was the crown of thorns, "the points of which were coming out [of her skin], and were touched by her Confessor."[53] The preponderance of well-documented and unusual physical details in this case should have invited medical evaluation. However, the local inquisitors dismissed the case without a medical investigation. They stated their reasons for denying the possibility of her sanctity and the superfluity of a medical examination: the tribunal thought that "a woman of so few years, and without the precedence of a long period of penance and a continual exercise of the most heroic virtues, is prevented from enjoying the privileges of the great saints Francis of Assisi and Catherine of Siena."[54] That is, bodily evidence only counted if the person experiencing the somatic signs already enjoyed an approved fame of sanctity that had been attested to by long years of holy behavior.[55] Anatomical evidence depended on context when it came to defining the boundaries of the supernatural.[56]

---

52   Biblioteca Nazionale di Roma, MS San Lorenzo in Lucina 60, f. 209 v. "Si vedevano spesse volte da suoi Confessori et altre Persone nelle di Lei mani, piedi, e lato sinistro le cicatrici rossegianti di sangue come se fosse state le stimmate della ricevuta passione."

53   Ibid., f. 210r: "procedesse d'alcune spine che p[ri]ma intorno alla d[ett]a piaga havevano cominciato ad uscire fuori con le punte, e toccate dal Confessore si sentivano inviscerate nella carne."

54   Ibid., f. 210v: "considerava il Tribunale parere non smosso in Termini di Santa, che una femina di cosi poca età, senza la precedenza d'una lunga penitenze e continuato esercizio delle più eroiche virtù fosse si toste prevenuta a godere i privilegii delli gran Santi Franc[esc]o d'Assisi o Catarina da Siena, ancorche con maggior prerogativa di quelli a quali non si erano mai vedute ne spine, ne chiodi et altre esterne visibili apparenze come di q[ues]ta si è detto." For more information about this fascinating case and the particulars of pretense of holiness in Sicily at this moment, see Gaetano Nicastro, *Donne e demoni nel Seicento: Un processo dell'inquisizione siciliana* (Acireale, 1990). I would like to thank Maria Pia Donato for pointing me to this helpful reference.

55   The argument that bodily evidence was considered much more suspect if it especially came from "little women," i.e. non-elite females, is a phenomenon that has been discussed elsewhere in the historical literature. See Schutte, *Aspiring Saints*, 42-60.

56   For additional discussion of the context of late seventeenth-century skepticism of female religiosity, see Marilena Modica, *Esperienza religiosa e scritture femminili tra medioevo ed età moderna* (Acireale, 1992).

This attitude of unwillingness to consider the possibility of physical signs of sanctity appears in numerous cases before the Inquisition in the seventeenth century. In Naples in 1629, for example, the various adherents to the cult of Andrea Castaldi, a Theatine monk, tried to encourage this cult by displaying prominently his supposedly incorrupt corpse.[57] Also in Naples, Andrea Avellino's body was widely reported to experience continued blood flow for years after his death in 1608, lasting until 1620.[58]

Several other cases from Rossano in Calabria, Beneventum, and Reggio all included physical evidence as part of the promotion of a local holy person's cult.[59] Each of these cases survives in the written record because the veneration of these unusual physical attributes was denounced to the Roman Inquisition, which then investigated and recorded it. Nevertheless, in none of these cases, which began due to the physical evidence that inspired veneration, was a medical professional called to evaluate the body.

Since in some of these cases the individual was later made a saint (e.g. Andrea Avellino), it was certainly not just the rank or gender of the person that prevented physical evidence being employed by the Inquisition. Rather, by the time cases reached the Inquisition there was already some concern that the veneration was excessive and unapproved in some way. The Inquisition's goal was, therefore, to slow or halt the veneration. Calling a physician or other well-known local medical practitioner might have backfired and drawn more attention to this case.

That the Inquisition was concerned about calling on expert medical witnesses because the action might encourage veneration of non-canonized, but locally venerated holy people, comes out clearly in a slightly later case that was documented in Ancona in 1710. In that year a priest noticed a "most pleasing odor, coming from a tomb."[60] He asked for and received permission from the bishop to open the tomb to search for the source of the odor. This led to the discovery of a body that seemed to have been buried for a number of years, yet that had resisted rot in a wondrous way and smelled wonderfully. The only problem was that no one knew the identity of the deceased.[61]

---

57   ACDF, St. St. MS B-4-C, fasc. 12.

58   ACDF, St. St. MS B-4-B, fasc. 1, f. 38r; for a longer discussion of the Theatines' promotion of
      its own members through a variety of propaganda efforts, see Vittoria Fiorelli, "'Apparati,
      musichi e sermoni in lode di lui.' Il disciplinamento devozionale dei Teatini napoletani
      nel secolo XVII," in Domenico Antonio D'Alessandro, ed., Sant'Andrea Avellino e i Teatini
      nella Napoli del viceregno spagnolo (Naples, 2011), 251-272.

59   ACDF, St. St. MS B-4-B, fasc. 14; ACDF, St. St. MS B-4-F, fasc. 1; ACDF, St. St. MS B-4-P, fasc. 3.

60   ACDF, St. St. MS B-4-P, fasc. 13, p. 1: "che scopertosi da un Prete di Cingoli [...] un gratissimo
      odore, che esalava da una sepoltura."

61   ACDF, St. St. MS B-4-P, fasc. 13, p. 4. The record asserts that it might have been the body of

As excitement built around this anonymous incorrupt corpse, the bishop of the nearby diocese of Osimo stepped in and took over the investigation. The Bishop of Osimo was not any provincial ecclesiastic, but Michelangelo dei Conti, the future Pope Innocent XIII (r. 1721-1724). By 1710 dei Conti held doctorates in canon and civil law, was a cardinal, had served as governor in a number of important posts in the Papal States, and had been appointed bishop of Osimo in the previous year. That is, he was an eminent ecclesiastical official with longstanding experience in dealing with a variety of political and religious matters.

Dei Conti began documenting what occurred in this investigation and sent several letters to the Roman Inquisition explaining what he was undertaking.[62] Perhaps trying to maintain a discreet distance between a canonization proceeding and an inquisition trial, dei Conti quietly organized a visit to the tomb. According to the record, he summoned two unnamed surgeons to judge "according to their art and their skill" whether there might be "some particular sign that is not currently present in the body, but which might arise in the bones" that would provide a key to the person's identity.[63] The surgeons in this case, though, were asked to proceed "with the greatest secrecy possible."[64] They were not asked for their opinion on whether the body could be considered miraculously incorrupt, or what the source of the odor might have been.

The facts that the surgeons remained anonymous in the record, that they were asked to proceed secretly, and that they were even then not questioned about whether the preservation was miraculous, but just whether they could tell the identity of the deceased, all suggest that dei Conti, and by extension the Inquisition officials with whom he was corresponding, did not want to publicize the use of medical expertise in this case. In several canonization trials the involvement of a medical professional in judging incorruption added a great deal of prestige to a prospective saint's cult, even if the judgment was ambigu-

---

Alessandro Ilarione: "Per cominciare assertione di tenevea [sic] che de[tto] cadavere forse di Alessandro Ilarione Pitto[r]e Rom[an]o." Elsewhere it asserts that this was a fiction (fasc. 13, p. 1): "che si pretendeva esser d'un tale Alessandro Ilarione Pittore Romano."

62   ACDF, St. St. MS B-4-P, fasc. 13, p. 1.

63   ACDF, St. St. MS B-4-P, fasc. 13, second document, p. 3. "Et se nel disseppellirlo c'avessero addotto qualche segno particolare, che presentemente non apparisse nel cadavere, ma potessa risultare dall'ossa; sotto porra' all'essami dei Periti chirurghi per procurare di verificarlo mediante le diligenzi da farsi dalli med. secondo la loro arte, et peritia."

64   ACDF, St. St. MS B-4-P, fasc. 13, second document, p. 1: "con la maggior segretezza possibile fare giudizialm[en]te l'accesso alla d[ett]a sepoltura."

ous or negative.[65] It may have been with this in mind that dei Conti decided to scrupulously avoid bringing in prestigious medical professionals. He needed medical skill to help identify the body, but feared the effect of excessive attention, which might encourage veneration of this anonymous corpse. In the end, the surgeons could not determine who the person was, and the body was re-buried quietly in another place so as to end the veneration.[66]

If the desire to avoid adding to the enthusiasm for a prospective saint's cult and the concern about the person's qualities were two central reasons why inquisitors tended not to ask medical professionals for their opinions in cases of possible false sanctity, another factor was the high cost of hiring physicians to perform these tasks. After examining the financial records of the office of the Roman Inquisition in Ferrara, Adriano Prosperi has determined that regional branches of the Inquisition operated on budgets as small as 82 *lire* a year.[67] However, the Congregation of Rites regularly paid medical experts who testified during canonization proceedings the high rate of ten *scudi* for a written statement and three *scudi* for deposing in person. Multiple testimonies might result in multiple payments.[68] It is likely that the Inquisition would have had to pay comparable rates for expert medical witnesses in its proceedings, since the nature of the testimony and expertise would have been similar. Although relative currency values fluctuated, a papal *scudo* was generally worth more than a *lira* in this period, so paying for one medical testimony would have been more than ten percent of the annual budget for most regional branches of the Roman Inquisition. A reason why inquisitors did not seek out medical expertise more frequently, then, may simply have been that they could not afford it.

That being said, financial considerations were not a determining factor everywhere that the Roman Inquisition operated. The central tribunal of the Inquisition in Rome regularly kept medical professionals on retainer. Giovanni Tiracorda, for example, an eminent Roman physician who also worked at the Santo Spirito Hospital and trained Giovanni Maria Lancisi, among others, was employed by the Roman Inquisition for twenty years.[69] He received a salary of twenty-five *scudi* annually for his services. When he died, there were numerous

---

65   Bradford Bouley, "Negotiated Sanctity: Incorruption, Community, and Medical Expertise," *The Catholic Historical Review*, 102, No. 1 (2016), 19-23; Laura Smoller, *The Saint and the Chopped-Up Baby* (Ithaca, NY, 2014), 50-54; 82-84.

66   ACDF, St. St. MS B-4-P, fasc. 13, p. 1: "facesse riposta d[ett]o Cadavere in altro luogo segreto."

67   Adriano Prosperi, "Il 'budget' di un inquisitore: Ferrara 1567-1572," in idem, *L'Inquisizione romana: Letture e ricerche* (Rome, 2003), 125-140.

68   Benedict XIV, *De servorum Dei beatificatione et beatorum canonizatione liber tertius* (Bologna, 1737), 426, 588.

69   ACDF, *Oeconomica* 6, ff. 15r, 33r, 38v, 46v, 59r, 282v-282r, and numerous other occurrences

applications to be his replacement, with Domenico Gerosi eventually securing the position.[70] But what did these medical practitioners do to earn their retainer from the Roman Inquisition?

In general, it would seem that physicians on retainer with the Roman Inquisition checked on the health of those detained by the Inquisition. One letter from the records of the Inquisition comes from the director of the Hospice of the Convertendi in Rome, a domicile in which Protestants could stay while converting to the Catholic faith. The director asked that the Inquisition allow medical examinations of the prospective converts, because there were several that were ill. If the Inquisition's physicians determined that there was a "dangerous sickness," the patient would be allowed to move more quickly through the Catholic rites so that they could enter into the fold of the faithful before dying.[71]

In another example, in 1692 the Inquisition's physician, Domenico Gerosi, found that several of the inmates imprisoned by the Inquisition were suffering from regular headaches. He suspected that the problem was caused by the construction taking place near their windows, which prevented the flow of fresh air.[72] He petitioned for and received the right to have the prisoners moved until the construction was over.[73] The Inquisition's account books show several payments to apothecaries with the express note that the purchased items would be used for the incarcerated. In 1653, for example, the apothecary Granduzzi seems to have been on retainer, as he received ninety-five *scudi* "for medical items given to the associates and prisoners of the Holy Office during the past year."[74] In short, the evidence suggests that the medical practitioners on retainer with the Inquisition were concerned with the health of the incarcerated and the employees of the Inquisition, but were not ever consulted about matters related to the actual business of the Inquisition. This finding agrees with Federico Barbierato's research on the Venetian Inquisition, where he has found that physicians employed by the Inquisition were normally tasked only with assessing the health of prisoners, and generally whether they were fit to stand trial.[75]

---

in this document. On Tiracorda, see Gaetano Marini, *Degli archiatri pontifici,* vol. 1 (Rome, 1784), xliii.

70   ACDF, *Privilegi S. officii urbis 1669-1699* (hereafter *Privilegi*), f. 702r.

71   Ibid., ff. 698r-699v.

72   Ibid., f. 708r.

73   Ibid., f. 709v.

74   ACDF, *Oeconomia* 6, ff. 8r, 18v: "di robbe medicinali date per la famiglia e carcerati del S. Offitto per tutto l'anno passatto."

75   Federico Barbierato, "Il medico e l'inquisitore: Note su medici e perizie mediche nel tribu-

In summary, then, the relationship between the Roman Inquisition and medical expertise presents a possible counterpoint to recent studies that have demonstrated the cooperation between medical expertise and church authority in understanding the natural world.[76] The Inquisition refused to use medical criteria to evaluate whether or not evidence of bodily abnormality was divinely or demonically inspired. The decision to discount medical expertise in this way, though, was not based on any failure to recognize the achievements and value of medicine for understanding the natural world. Indeed, most of the inquisitors would have been very familiar with the attempts to use medical evidence in a variety of ecclesiastical contexts.[77] Rather, the reticence to use medicine can, in a way, be attributed to early modern success of medicine. Involving a physician might bring unwanted attention to a case that the inquisitors were attempting to slow or even quash. Furthermore, consulting such expertise could be costly and might add little to a case where the verdict had already been determined by other social and cultural factors, such as the gender and social status of the accused. Whatever the reason, though, the Roman Inquisition's decision not to employ medicine in the discernment of spirits would seem to mirror more current attitudes concerning the relationship between medicine and belief. Although the achievements of medicine were respected, it had no place in evaluating the spirituality of a person accused by the Inquisition of false sanctity. That is, science and religion seemed to inhabit different spheres – an idea that many in the Western world would take as the natural relationship between the two, but which was by no means the dominant view in the seventeenth century.[78]

---

nale del Sant'Uffizio veneziano fra Sei e Settecento," in Pastore and Rossi, eds., *Paolo Zacchia*, 266-285.

76   Elisa Andretta, *Anatomie du vénérable dans la Rome de la contre-réforme: Les autopsies d'Ignace de Loyola et de Philippe Neri*, in Maria Pia Donato and Jill Kraye, eds., *Conflicting Duties: Science, Medicine and Religion in Rome, 1550-1750* (London, 2009), 255-280; Bouley, *Pious Postmortems*; Nancy Siraisi, "Signs and Evidence: Autopsy and Sanctity in Late Sixteenth-Century Italy," *Medicine and the Italian Universities, 1250-1600* (Boston, MA, 2001), 356-380. For more general discussions of the relationship between medicine and religion in this period, see Maria Pia Donato, "Medicina e religione: Percorsi di lettura," in Maria Pia Donato et al., eds., *Médecine et religion: Collaborations, competitions, conflits (XIIe-XXe siècles)* (Rome, 2013), 11-33; Rivka Feldhay, "Religion," in Katharine Park and Lorraine Daston, eds., *The Cambridge History of Science*, vol. 3, *Early Modern Science* (New York, NY, 2006), 727-755.

77   See above, note 19.

78   Feldhay, "Religion," 727-730; Amos Funkenstein, *Theology and the Scientific Imagination from the Middle Ages to the Seventeenth Century* (Princeton, NJ, 1986), 346.

Anatomy of a Scandal: Physicians Facing the Inquisition in Late Seventeenth-Century Rome

Maria Pia Donato
CNRS, Institut d'Histoire Moderne et Contemporaine
mpdonato@alice.it

Abstract

In the 1690s the Roman Inquisition targeted medical circles, as they allegedly disseminated atheism under the veil of new explanations of the body. This article revisits these affairs, focussing on Rome. It argues that increased inquisitorial pressure must be set against the backdrop of struggles for hegemony in the papal curia, in which physicians were entangled. Notwithstanding such political vicissitudes, ecclesiastical control played a relevant role in shaping Italian medicine at the turn of the seventeenth and eighteenth centuries. The article suggests that the result may have been, paradoxically, a form of un-assumed materialism, though framed within the disciplinary borders of practical medicine, which enabled physicians to re-assert their autonomy.

Keywords

atomism – medicine and religion – free-thinking – Cartesianism – Giovanni M. Lancisi – medical ethics – Inquisition – mechanical medicine

In the 1690s medical circles were targeted on by the Roman Inquisition, as they allegedly disseminated atheism and scepticism under the veil of new explanations of the body and nature. Even in Rome, prominent physicians were put on trial on suspicion of atheism, and a medical academy was disbanded. Was this a flagrant confirmation of the old dictum, *tres medici, duo athei*?

*   Ecole Normale Supérieure, 45, rue d'Ulm, 75005, Paris, France. I would like to express my gratitude to Bradford Bouley and the anonymous referees for their useful comments. This article is dedicated to the memory of Elena Brambilla (1942-2018).

In what follows, my aim is to revisit the trials against physicians in the light of old and new archival evidence. I will augment this evidence by drawing on the growing body of scholarship on the Roman Church and the Inquisition, which has highlighted their internal fractures and the contingent nature of dogma. The focus of this essay will be Rome, which, as the seat of the Holy Office and the papacy, provides a good vantage point for observing medical practitioners in their social environment and vis-à-vis ecclesiastical control.

In recent years, some scholars have argued that modern natural philosophy, and especially atomism, implied the spread of atheism among medical practitioners, to which the Inquisition reacted.[1] While making new sources available, these studies reintroduce a fixist understanding of free-thinking in opposition to 'orthodoxy,' and disregard the complexities of the early-modern physician's social persona.[2] I will argue that increased inquisitorial pressure must, in fact, be set against a backdrop of struggles for hegemony in the papal curia and shifts in Catholic spirituality. The late seventeenth-century Inquisition was a complex institution that acted in the context of an unstable set of circumstances. Physicians were part of an intricate, politically mobile, socially mixed world; in an age of rapid change in medical practice and theory they were caught in factional clashes that coalesced both on theology and natural philosophy. Given the complexity of these conflicts, only micro-historical cases like that of the 'atheist' physicians in 1690 Rome discussed here can shed light on the intertwining of these different aspects.

This does not imply that ecclesiastical control did not play a role in shaping medicine. First, the Inquisition periodically re-enacted the subordination of lay intellectuals to ecclesiastics, while underpinning social hierarchies. Furthermore, the collapse of Aristotelianism and Galenism created friction at the margins of the distinct, although overlapping, fields of medicine, philosophy and metaphysics, which the Inquisition sought to police. In a ground-breaking article of 1984, Elena Brambilla noted that, due to inquisitorial control, eighteenth-century Italian medicine was characterised by an inductive method pertaining only to the description of nature as it was

---

1 See, e.g., Candida Carella, *Roma filosofica nicodemita libertina: Scienza e censura in età moderna* (Lugano, 2014); and especially Vittorio Frajese, *Dal libertinismo ai Lumi: Roma 1690–Torino 1727* (Rome, 2017).

2 For a critical reassessment of libertinism and the pitfalls of criminal records, see Jean-Pierre Cavaillé, "Le 'libertinage érudit': Fertilité et limites d'une catégorie historiographique," *Les Dossiers du Grihl* 2011 (<http://dossiersgrihl.revues.org/4827>, accessed 3 March 2018); Thomas Berns, Anne Staquet and Monique Weis, eds., *Libertin! Usages d'une invective aux XVIe et XVIIe siècles* (Paris, 2013).

visible to the naked eye.[3] Here it is argued that the result was, paradoxically, a form of un-assumed materialism, though carefully framed within the disciplinary confines of practical medicine.

Filing Accusations Against 'Atheist' Physicians

In August 1690, a physician, Sulpizio Antonio Mazzuti, was arrested in Rome by armed officers of the Inquisition. The Holy Office had already been concerned about Mazzuti: some months previously, during the Vacant Seat following Innocent XI's death, he had spontaneously confessed to having read prohibited books *ad artem medicam spectantes*. Owning prohibited books without a licence and confessing it spontaneously during the Vacant See, when one could easily get clemency, was common practice, especially among university-trained doctors who were expected to be aware of the state of the art.[4] Yet, the allegations were now serious: he was deemed an atheist who cursed Jesus and the Apostles, denied the existence of miracles, and believed that "all things are made by accident."[5]

Mazzutti's arrest was part of a bigger affair, involving a "sect" of free-thinkers allegedly plotting against the papal government. The leader of these *Bianchi*, as they called themselves, was a young noble prelate, Pietro Gabrielli, who was already notorious for his provocative attitude, which went beyond what was tolerated at the court of Rome. Testimonies describe a party of young men of different social statuses (an apothecary, a musician, a clerk, and a simple handyman, all apprehended) inclined towards wine, women and iconoclasm, who debated religion and politics.[6] Sometimes they delved into nature's se-

---

3 Elena Brambilla, "La medicina del Settecento: Dal monopolio dogmatico alla professione scientifica," in Franco Della Perruta, ed., *Storia d'Italia,* Annali 7, *Malattia e medicina* (Turin, 1984), 5-147, 27.

4 Archivio della Congregazione per la Dottrina della Fede (henceforth ACDF), *Decreta Sancti Officii*, 1689, f. 307v. The ownership of prohibited books was common among elite physicians, see for instance Fabiola Zurlini, *Romolo Spezioli (Fermo, 1642 – Roma, 1723): Un medico fermano a Roma nel XVII secolo* (Manziana, 2000). On licences for medical books, see Ugo Baldini and Leen Spruit, *Catholic Church and Modern Science: Documents from the Archives of the Roman Congregations of the Holy Office and the Index,* part 1: *The Sixteenth Century* (Rome, 2009).

5 ACDF, St. St. O3f, f. 294v.

6 The heretical propositions recorded in ACDF, St. St. UV6, feature a mixture of learned references to classic atheistic *topoi*, ancient and modern Epicureism, and popular anticlericalism. On the Bianchi, see Giorgio Spini, *Ricerca dei libertini* (Florence, 1983), 355-367; Dalma Frascarelli and Laura Testa, *La casa dell'eretico: Arte e cultura nella quadreria romana di Pietro*

crets with an elderly underworld philosopher, Antonio Oliva. A former member of the Cimento academy, Oliva now lived in Rome, healing with his secret medicines under the protection of Lorenzo Onofrio Colonna, the Grand Connetable of Naples, and a patron of the arts notoriously interested in alchemy. Oliva was accused of denying Creation and transubstantiation in the Eucharist, "a thing impossible and against nature's first principles."[7]

The inquisitors, who were used to dealing with unruly noblemen, were inclined to think that all these 'atheists' were hot-minded youngsters.[8] Nonetheless, the strong political and anti-clerical undertone made the matter serious, especially because the lower classes were involved.

Following Gabrielli and Mazzuti's arrest, accusations snowballed. On August 12, the former papal archiater, Giovanni M. Lancisi, presented himself to the Inquisition. He admitted that in his youth he had read prohibited books by authors like Machiavelli, Sextus Empiricus, and Erasmus, "with the aim of making himself learned and fashionable." This had given him "false and despicable opinions," but he claimed to have found the light of truth again after he had been appointed physician to the late Pope Innocent XI and read the Fathers; Mazzutti, by contrast, was an unbeliever, spreading things contrary to religion and "showing the imposture, that is, that we have to believe the mysteries of the Faith out of ignorance."[9]

Some days later, a man of lower condition, Giovan Francesco Bolla, having heard that "sects of atheists were being searched," reported that a few years

---

Gabrielli (1660-1734) a Palazzo Taverna di Montegiordano (Rome, 2004), where the documents are partly published. On unbelief as a socially pervasive phenomenon, see Nicholas Davidson, "Unbelief and Atheism in Italy, 1500-1700," in Michael Hunter and David Wotton, eds., *Atheism from the Reformation to the Enlightenment* (Oxford, 1992), 55-85.

7   ACDF, St. St. UV6, f. 122r-v, hearing of Filippo Alfonsi: "Che il sacramento dell'Eucharestia era una cosa impossibile, e contro i primi principi naturali." On Oliva, see Ugo Baldini, *Un libertino accademico del Cimento, Antonio Oliva* (Florence, 1977). On Colonna, see Elena Tamburini, *Due teatri per il principe: Studi sulla committenza teatrale di Lorenzo Onofrio Colonna (1659-1689)* (Rome, 1997); Natalia Gozzano, *La quadreria di Lorenzo Onofrio Colonna: Prestigio nobiliare e collezionismo nella Roma barocca* (Rome, 2004).

8   ACDF, St. St. UV6, ff. 180r-183r. The Inquisition repeatedly received denunciations against young noblemen for their provocative behaviour, see, e.g., ACDF, St. St. I4i, unnumberd ff., against Lelio Carandini.

9   ACDF, St. St. UV60, n° 40, published by Carella, *Roma*, 143-152, here 144-145, "al fine di farsi erudito e dotarsi d'un buon stile"; "un embrione confuso d'opinioni false e detestabili"; "mostrava l'impostura, cioè che a noi veniva imposta la credenza de misteri della medesima fede per nostra ignoranza." Notably, this is a summary of the trial drawn up in the 1730s by the Inquisition's assessor or archivist, as was customary at the time; the original trial records are now lost, as is the overwhelming majority of the Holy Office's criminal records.

previously Lancisi had been his family's physician; that he told his sister-in-law Chiara, whom he courted, that the soul died with the body, hell did not exist, and saints and miracles were mere fables. Bolla also reported that Lancisi scandalized the women he cured boasting his own superior education.[10] Chiara Bolla and her mother-in-law themselves were interrogated. They maintained their accusations and expressed disbelief that such a "light-minded, vain pedant" had risen to the position of papal doctor.[11]

Having been alerted that accusations were still pending, on September 6, Lancisi gave a second testimony. He claimed that Chiara was retaliating because he had left her to take up the post of papal physician. But he now acknowledged that he had debated religious problems with Mazzuti and others of higher status and in the curial milieu (including Angelo del Noce, an erudite prelate in the entourage of Christine of Sweden), and even with women. Lancisi's defence consisted in pointing out the conflicting obligations of university-trained physicians: to show his wit and learning, he claimed, he had debated the eternity of the world, positing that this would make Divine Providence superfluous, because all that "make up the world, whether seeds, organs or principles of mouvement" would move by itself; and he had also wondered whether the perfection of the human soul depended on the perfection of the body – as Galen had taught, a classic problem that had engaged many physicians (famously Huarte de San Juan).[12] However, he insisted that his motive had always been to "show erudition, not for any belief contrary to the Faith."[13]

In the meantime, fearing to be involved himself, Albert Gunther (italianized Ganteri), a 57-year old German physician from the Catholic enclave of Mainz who had graduated in 1659 and had been practicing in Rome for some years, pointed his finger at the entire circle of *novatores*. For some time he had taken part in an academy, the *Congresso medico,* which met every Monday in the house of the doctor Girolamo Brasavola with the aim of debating classic medical problems in the light of new doctrines. Gunther reported that the academy harboured "maxims and principle of atomist philosophers."[14] His testimony

10 Carella, *Roma*, 143-144, "che si sveglino queste sette di ateisti."

11 Carella, *Roma,* 148, "leggiero vanarello e dottorino."

12 Ibid., 149: "per mostrare bell'ingegno"; "tutte le parti componenti del mondo, che fossero semi, organi, e principij di moto non vi era bisgono della providenza di Dio, perche da se stesse si moverebbero, e continuarebbero le vicende, le mutationi, e quelle che si chiamano generationi"; "che la perfetioni ch'haveva detta anima sopra gl'altri animali, potevano dervare dalla perfettione degl'organi, ch'haveva sopra gl'altri animali."

13 Ibid., p. 151, "per mostrare erudizione, e non per credenza contraria alla fede."

14 ACDF, St. St. O1n, n° 10, f. 295r: "questi congressi accademici si facevano infallibilmente una volta la settimana cioè il lunedì sera. In questa accademia uno discorreva sopra

was confused, as he remembered the names of few academicians, but reported that Lancisi and Mazzuti were followers of Epicurus, Gassendi and Descartes. He recalled that they had been vocal in defending Descartes (whose *opera* had been suspended by the Index in 1663). The inquisitors hence started a further dossier against Lancisi, Brasavola, Giacomo Sinibaldi and Domenico Gerosi on the grounds that they had claimed that "everything was made of the casual movement of atoms through their position, shape and configuration," and "intellect, measure, position and movement of atoms are inherent in matter since the beginning of things."[15]

Policing Medical Practice for a Catholic Society

In many regards, this minor *inquisitio* of 1690 is emblematic of the control that the Inquisition, and more broadly the Catholic Church, sought to exert on medical practitioners. Because physicians shared their patients' precarious moments in life, they were suspect, as they could induce frail persons into error, sin and even heresy, instead of contributing to their spiritual redemption, as they were supposed to.[16]

The sixteenth-century Inquisition was primarily concerned with Protestant propaganda, and medical practitioners were often investigated for converting others to Evangelism.[17] After the fear of a Lutheran 'infection' subsided, ecclesiastical authorities continued to consider physicians as potentially dangerous. Unfortunately, the fragmentary condition of diocesan and collegiate archives, both in Rome and in other Italian cities, along with the loss of the Holy Office criminal records makes it difficult to assess how many practitioners were reprimanded for 'catechizing' their patients into erroneous beliefs. Nevertheless, the fact that a steady flow of literature that was produced to remind practitioners that medicine was subordinate to religion suggests that the Church fought

---

qualche punto filosofico e medicinale a suo beneplacito, e poscia si risolveva una questione cavata a sorte da due accademici, ed in detti discorsi più volte ho sentito discorrere la dottrina degl'atomi secondo l'insegnamento di Cartesio, Cassendo e Epicuro."

15   Ibid., f. 294v: "quod omnia generatur ex causalis et fortuito atomorum concursu, ex vario situ, positura et configuratione et ulterius quod mens, mensura, quies, motus, positura, figura sint ad materia ab exordio rerum." See Maria Pia Donato, "L'onere della prova: Il Sant'Uffizio, l'atomismo e i medici romani," *Nuncius: Annali di storia della scienza*, 18 (2003), 69-87.

16   Alessandro Pastore, *Le regole dei corpi: Medicina e disciplina nell'Italia moderna* (Bologna, 2006).

17   See Alessandra Celati's article in this volume.

a restless battle against religiously ambiguous medics. Physicians were considered the quintessential worldly men of learning who sacrificed scruples on the altar of fame, fortune, and fashion. Indeed, devotional books often rebuked them for their lax piety.[18]

Allegations against Mazzuti and Lancisi fit into such a pattern, and all the more so as they included claims of sexual misconduct, another problematic area of the doctor-patient relationship. Throughout Catholic Europe, medical practitioners were in the overwhelming majority lay persons, hence mostly (sooner or later) married men – family connections were, in fact, crucial for a successful career. Yet in Rome, unmarried physicians were held in esteem and were granted some privileges, like accessing ecclesiastical benefices and living in the Vatican Palaces if appointed physician to the pope. Likewise, only unmarried young doctors could enter into an internship in the main city hospital of Santo Spirito in Sassia. This implied that there were many single practitioners, like Lancisi himself, who were easily liable to claims of sexual misconduct. A few years previously, Florindo Salvatori, the papal physician and *Protomedicus*, was convicted of rape, stripped of his canonicate, and held in jail before he was rehabilitated.[19]

Furthermore, because they treated different kinds of people, physicians were at the intersection of various social worlds, and were inherently at risk of short-circuiting social codes. Libertinism (especially uttering a certain disdain for the beliefs of the simple minded) was not uncommon in Rome among the elites.[20] This mark of social distinction was possible, provided that one had the right protectors in the right milieu; by contrast, to get above one's status thanks to one's wit could stir resentment in the lower classes. In the 1690 events under discussion here, physicians acted between the popular environment, the curial underworld, nobility, and the court, but apparently infringed the moral expectations of each.

Yet the affair went beyond the disciplining pattern of medical practice and the hint of unbelief that stigmatized the medical profession in the eyes of clerics. In fact, allegations against Lancisi and his colleagues touched upon specific philosophical issues, namely atomism, thus raising the problem of the

---

18　See, e.g., Daniello Bartoli, *La ricreazione del savio in discorso con la natura e con Dio* (Rome, 1659); idem, *L'huomo al punto cioè l'huomo in punto di morte* (Rome, 1667), 197-222, 316-324; Jean Crasset, *La douce et sainte mort* (Lyon, 1681).

19　Filippo M. Renazzi, *Storia dell'Università di Roma*, vol. 3 (Rome, 1805), 191.

20　Dalma Frascarelli, ed., *L'altro Seicento: Arte a Roma tra eterodossia, libertinismo e scienza* (Rome, 2016).

ecclesiastical censorship of natural philosophy, its antecedents and context, to
which it is now necessary to turn.

Portrait of the Physician as a Virtuoso

In the final decades of the seventeenth century, criticism of Aristotelian and
scholastic philosophy was voiced increasingly loudly in Rome. Echoing similar
debates that emerged in other parts of Italy and Europe, learned prelates and
virtuosi engaged in an overt discussion of atomism as an alternative to Aristotelian principles, which no longer seemed compatible with Christianity.[21] The
pontificates of Clement IX and Innocent XI seem to have offered a particularly
favourable context. Pope Innocent XI was notoriously hostile to the Jesuits. He
favoured ecclesiastical erudition and positive theology, which necessarily involved some degree of anti-scholasticism, and he also intended to curtail the
Inquisition's prerogatives. His attitudes left open room for philosophical speculation about science and medicine, and what authorities should actually be
relied on.

For medicine too, the time had come to explicitly rebut Galen's ideas of faculties and souls. Spectacular demonstrations of modern circulatory physiology
were staged, and problematic aspects of the Galenic-Aristotelian heritage –
movement, sensation and generation – came under scrutiny.[22] Some drew
upon a dynamic Sennertian and Gassendian corpuscularism.[23] Others, like
Lucantonio Porzio, a Neapolitan physician teaching in Rome, combined mechanism and atomistic matter theories.[24] But it is difficult (and ultimately irrele-
vant) to draw a divide between a mechanical and a chemical-qualitative
approach. Giovanni Alfonso Borelli is a case in point. He lived in Rome in the
final years of his life under the patronage of Queen Christina of Sweden, com-

21   Craig Martin, *Subverting Aristotle: Religion, History, and Philosophy in Early Modern Sci-
      ence* (Baltimore, MD, 2014).

22   See, e.g., Paolo Manfredi, *Ragguaglio degl'esperimenti ... circa la nuova operatione della
      trasfusione del sangue da individuo ad individuo, ed in bruti ed in huomini* (Rome, 1668);
      idem, *Novae circa aurem observationes* (Rome, 1674); idem, *Novae circa oculum observatio-
      nes* (Rome, 1674); Caspar Bartholin, *De ovariis mulierum et generationis historia* (Rome,
      1677); Domenico Gagliardi, *Anatome ossium* (Rome, 1989).

23   Gregorio Roscio, *Rerum naturalium cogitationes*, MS Rome, Biblioteca Alessandrina, 191.

24   Lucantonio Porzio, *In Hippocratis librum de veteri medicina ... paraphrasis* (Rome, 1681),
      on which see Alessandro Dini, *Filosofia della natura, medicina, religione: Lucantonio
      Porzio (1639-1724)* (Milan, 1985).

pleting his *On the Motion of Animals*. When the book appeared in 1680 it featured a mixture of mechanical philosophy and corpuscularianism.[25]

Faculty members, especially the younger ones, and physicians at court were eager to distinguish themselves by showing their support for modern tenets. It was precisely the goal of academies like the Congresso to be particularly visible in the professional arena while increasing the cultural acceptance of contemporary medical theories. In Rome too, Galenism was in the process of becoming a synonym for useless therapeutic conservatism.[26] As Sinibaldi himself would later write with some degree of oversimplification, Galenism was challenged by a "very new sect of our times that follows the dogmas of Descartes, or Atomists."[27] Even surgeons upheld ideas of circulatory physiology and corpuscular philosophy, and preferred now to "speak with Descartes" and consider the body as a clockwork.[28]

The four practitioners accused by the inquisition in 1690 are representative of such a shift in the theoretical assumptions and ideological posture of Roman medicine, and were fully engaged in new medical ideas.

Girolamo Brasavola, in whose house the group used to meet, was a descendant of the illustrious humanist Antonio Musa, and had graduated from Ferrara; in Rome, he was in the service of cardinal Carlo Pio of Savoy, and the primary doctor at the Santo Spirito hospital. In 1655 and 1676 he had been the conclave's doctor. In his lectures, Brasavola claimed to reconcile Gassendi, Van Helmont, Willis and Descartes, and taught that matter was formed by corpuscles or *semina* endowed with movement by God. All transformations in nature happened through fermentation, which by 'weakening' the form of corpuscles enabled them to be transformed in mixes and aggregates. All operations in the body happened through fermentation thanks to ferments secreted by the various organs.[29] In the early 1680s Brasavola promoted the *Congresso medico*, which rapidly gained fame (it enjoyed the protection of no fewer than six car-

---

25   Giovanni Alfonso Borelli, *De motu animalium* (Rome, 1680-81). Book Two, in particular, delves into movements on a micro-analytical level, and combines a mechanical and chemical understanding of corpuscles, which Borelli endowed with *vis plastica* in explaining generation. See further Francesco Spoleti, *De secretione bilis in hepate* (Venice, 1686).

26   Vivian Nutton, *The Fortunes of Galen*, in Robert J. Hunkinson, ed., *The Cambridge Companion to Galen* (Cambridge, 2008), 355-390, 378.

27   Giacomo Sinibaldi, *Institutiones medicinae theoricae*, London, Wellcome Library, MS 4182, f. 7r, "novissima secta nostris temporis [...] sequens Chartesii dogmata, seu Athomistarum" (the manuscript, undated, probably dates from the early 1700s).

28   Bernardino Genga, *Anatomia chirurgica* (Rome, 1686), 308, See further Mario Cecchini, *Elenchus lectionum et ostentionum ... in theatro anatomico ... S. Iacobi* (Rome, 1683-1688).

29   Federica Favino, "Sostanza e materia in uno scritto inedito di Girolamo Brasavola," *Medicina nei secoli*, 15 (2003), 247-267.

dinals), and he appeared to continue favouring chemical notions.[30] In 1684 he was promoted to the position of chief physician to the papal household.

Sinibaldi was born in Rome. He was the son and brother of prominent physicians, and received his doctorate in 1659. He was a lecturer in *materia medica* and a proponent of chemical medicine, and made his students defend theses such as "the elements are five, salt, sulphur, spiritus, water and earth," and "there is no need to suppose the first matter of Aristotelians."[31] In the Congresso, Sinibaldi supported Willis' mechanical-chemical theory of fermentation as an alternative to the Galenic aetiology of fever. Speaking on insect generation, he posited that it was produced by the fermentation of sulphur salts ignited by heat.[32] Sinibaldi later became the Chair of theoretical medicine, and in 1685 he entered the College of Physicians. In 1690, the very year of his inquisitorial misadventure, he published a collection of academic and university lectures, in which he maintained his preference for a mildly chemical medicine, and notably, for the work of Willis.[33]

Mazzuti graduated in Fermo in 1670, and was a protégé of his compatriot cardinal Decio Azzolino. His only printed work was a dissertation of 1684 on women's pathologies and hysteric frenzy, in which he claimed that all diseases originated from "the innumerable sorts of particles [...] which, if they are retained in the ocean of fluids, associate themselves in various, diverse ways, take diverse, various positions, and become the seed of multiples diseases."[34]

Not much is known of Domenico Gerosi, except that he was a protégé of an influential prelate, Lorenzo Corsini (later Pope Clement XII), and that he gained his doctorate in 1673, one year before Lancisi.

The latter, born in Rome, had been an assistant at the Santo Spirito. Since his student years he had been renowned for his command of ancient and modern

30   *Catalogo del Congresso medico romano: Ove sono descritti i nomi degli autori, e le materie da loro trattate ogni lunedì* (Rome, 1682); Girolamo Brasavola, *Problema an clysteres nutriant*, in *Congressus medico-romanus habitus in aedibus D. Hieronymi Brasavoli die lune 21. Septembris 1682* (Rome, 1682), 33-41.

31   [Giacomo Sinibaldi], *Embrio philosophicus sive Novum veteris philosophiae rudimentum XV propositionibus delineatum* (Rome, 1679), 5-7: "Elementa sunt quinque sal, sulphur, spiritus, aqua, terra ... Nulla est necessitas ponendi materiam primama Aristotelicorum."

32   Giacomo Sinibaldi, *Dell'abuso de' vescicatori, discorso* (Rome, 1681); *Congresso medico romano tenuto in casa del sig. d. Girolamo Brasavoli a dì 4 agosto 1687* (Rome, 1687), 4-16.

33   Idem, *Apollo Bifrons medicas et amoenas dissertationes ...* (Rome, 1690).

34   Sulpizio A. Mazzuti, *Historia medica coram eruditissimo doctorum coetu in aedibus Brasavolaeis Roma exposita* (Rome, 1685), 8, "innumera particularum genera [...] quae si in fluidorum oceano retineantur, varie, diverseque se invicem associantes, varias, diversasque positura sumunt, ac in multigena morborum semina abeunt."

medicine and philosophy.[35] He was very active in the Congresso. In 1684, he was appointed the lecturer of anatomy and surgery at the university, and taught that the human body was "a machine, not only mobile but self-moving, composed of innumerable and diverse solid little machines [...] and the fluids that flow therein."[36] Lancisi had wide-ranging interest in other areas of natural philosophy, too. He studied generation by observing fecundated chicken eggs through a microscope and subscribed to Malpighi's idea (which opposed Borelli's) that the ovum and the semen had infinitely little stamina that contributed to forming the embryo.[37] He was indeed a keen user of the microscope. Like *virtuosi* elsewhere in Europe, naturalists in Rome were fascinated by the prospect of establishing corpuscularianism experimentally; Lancisi forcefully claimed the usefulness of microscopes (which Galenists contested) for observing the "organic atoms" and the "most minute particles invisible to naked eye" caught in "that dark prison that ancient philosophers called the occult."[38] When in 1687 animalcules were observed in dog semen, Lancisi converted from ovism to animalculism.[39]

Lancisi also investigated religious frenzy from a medical perspective. In 1684 he discussed the story of a fasting virgin who vomited stones; following the teachings of Malpighi, he dismissed the possibility that the girl might be possessed or bewitched.[40] This kind of moderate scepticism was widespread

---

35 Lancisi's wide and diverse reading is attested to by his commonplace books or *Studia iuvenilia inchoata ab anno 1672 repertorium medicum,* MS Rome, Biblioteca Lancisiana (henceforth BL), Lancisi 193-214; Dalma Frascarelli, *L'arte del dissenso: Pittura e libertinismi nell'Italia del Seicento* (Turin, 2017), 93.

36 Giovanni M. Lancisi, "Anatomica humani corporis synopsis prolusio," in his *Opera varia,* vol. 2 (Venice, 1739), 78, "machinam non modo mobile, sed etiam se moventem, pluribus, diversisque, qua duris, qua mollibus, omnibus tam solidorum nomine venientibus machinulis coagmentatam una cum varies intercurrentibus [...] fluidis."

37 Idem, *Praelectiones de formatione foetus in utero,* MS Rome, BL, Lancisi 312, ff. 38r-56v.

38 MS Rome, BL, Lancisi 314, f. 36v, "essere i corpiccioli più minuti, e all'ochio nudo invisibili [...] i quali senza fallo restarebbero [...] racchiusi entro quel carcere profondo de filosofi antichi, detto, l'occulto, se da questa lente così picciola non fossero ingranditi quei, per così dire, atomi organici." See Christoph Meinel, "Early Seventeenth-Century Atomism: Theory, Epistemology, and the Insufficency of Experiment," *Isis,* 79 (1988), 68-103.

39 Walter Bernardi, *Le metafisiche dell'embrione: Scienze della vita e filosofia da Malpighi a Spallanzani* (Florence, 1986), 155-159.

40 *Congressus medico-romanus,* 3-10. On the naturalisation of bodily concretions, see Domenico Bertoloni Meli, "Blood, Monsters, and Necessity in Malpighi's *De polypo cordis,*" *Medical History,* 45 (2001), 511-522, and on wondrous fasting, Simon Schaffer, "Piety, Physic and Prodigious Abstinence," in Ole P. Grell and Andrew Cunningham, eds., *Religio medici: Medicine and Religion in Seventeenth-Century England* (Aldershot, 1996), 171-203; Walter

among rigorist Catholics who sought to purge faith of superstition by drawing upon natural philosophy and medicine. Finally, in 1688, aged 34, Lancisi was chosen as the papal archiater to Innocent XI. He moved to the Vatican and became a canon in the church of St Damasus (he did not, however, join the College of Physicians due to opposition from senior colleagues). Upon the death of the pope in 1689, as was customary, Lancisi performed the autopsy on the deceased, and then returned to teaching and private practice.[41]

Medicine, Politics and the Inquisition's Censorship of Natural Philosophy

In a nutshell, what the four practitioners introduced above had in common was that they had been eloquent in their allegiance to recent medicine, although each in his own way, and that they had enjoyed rather successful careers. By showcasing debates of atoms and corpuscles, and making them compatible with older ideas, the *Congresso medico* had served as a springboard for many members.

In the late 1680s, however, the context was no longer as favourable to explorations of man and nature, and to debates on the Christianization of atomism, as it had been in the preceding decades.

The Holy Office and the congregation of the Index actually looked upon contemporary physics, especially atomism, with increasing suspicion. I am not referring here to the censorship of medical works heralding corpuscular ideas, which from time to time attracted the attention of Roman censors alongside the incomparably more numerous devotional, theological, historical texts that kept them busy. For instance, Daniel Sennert's *Physica hypomnemata* was prohibited in 1639 on the grounds of his traducianism, whereas in the *Astronomiae microcosmicae systema novum* by a Neapolitan doctor, Sebastiano Bartoli, censors equated the Helmontian notion of *archeus* to a partial soul, and furthermore disapproved of Bartoli's virulent attacks on the Galenists.[42] Rather, the Inquisition's most significant perceived threats to religion in this period were posed by non-Aristotelian physics, particularly atomism, with its implications

Vandereycken and Ron van Deth, *From Fasting Saints to Anorexic Girls: The History of Self-Starvation* (London, 1994).

41   Lancisi, *Giornale dell'ultima infermità della S.M. di Innocenzo XI*, MS Rome, BL, Lancisi 148.

42   On Sennert, see ACDF, Index, *Protocolli* EE, ff. 19r-22r; Michael Stolberg, "Particles of the Soul: The Medical and Lutheran Context of Daniel Sennert's Atomism," *Medicina nei secoli*, 15 (2003), 177-203. On Bartoli, ACDF, Index, *Protocolli* OO, ff. 459r-460v.

for metaphysics. Of course, ancient atomism was already considered heretical in that it denied the Creation and the very existence of God. But rebuttals of Aristotelian substantial forms were now the focus of growing concern. This issue became particularly acute because corpuscularian explications of the Eucharist were spreading among theologians and triggered bitter controversies.[43] Such a clash led to the suspension of Descartes's work mentioned above.[44] In a crescendo of accusations that blended theological, moral and philosophical issues, the Holy Office eventually ordered local inquisitors to refuse to licence books which stated that "substantial composites are not made by matter and form but by atoms or corpuscles."[45]

It was not until the late 1680s, however, that the issue of 'modern philosophy' matured into a political as much as doctrinal question.[46] By then, a war in which theology, philosophy and politics intertwined had broken out. Tensions within the curia had escalated, and the Holy Office was attacking anything that could weaken the spiritual and cultural assets, including scholasticism, which underpinned the Counter-Reformation. An intransigent faction advocated for a firmer reaction to anything that jeopardized the prerogatives of the Inquisi-

---

43   The bibliography on this topic is now vast; see Pietro Redondi, *Galileo: Heretic* (Princeton, NJ, 1992); Massimo Bucciantini, *Contro Galileo: Alle origini dell'affaire* (Florence, 1995); Jean-Robert Armogathe, *Theologia cartesiana: L'explication physique de l'Eucharistie chez Descartes et dom Desgabets* (The Hague, 1977); Roger Ariew, *Descartes and the Late Scholastics* (Ithaca, NY, and London, 1999); Tad M. Schmaltz, *Radical Cartesianism: The French Reception of Descartes* (Cambridge, 2002).

44   It was in an effort to prove its orthodoxy that the pro-Jansenist Faculty of Louvain signalled the theological implications of Descartes' philosophy, whereas five years later, the *nuncio* in Paris described Gassendi's teachings as contrary to the Catholic faith, with the aim of discrediting the Jansenists. See, respectively, Jean-Robert Armogathe and Vincent Carraud, "La première condamnation de oeuvres de Descartes d'après les documents inédits aux archives du Saint-Office," *Nouvelles de la République des lettres*, 8 (2001), 103-123; Giuliano Gasparri, "Documenti dell'Archivio del Sant'Uffizio per servire alla storia del gassendismo in Italia (1668-1723)," *Nouvelles de la République des Lettres*, 28 (2008), 75-110, and more generally, Margaret J. Osler, "When Did Pierre Gassendi Become a Libertine?" in John Brooke and Ian Maclean, eds., *Heterodoxy in Science and Religion* (Oxford, 2005), 169-192.

45   "Composita substantialia non componitur ex materia, et forma, sed ex corpusculis seu atomis," in Donato, "L'onere," 69.

46   Maria Pia Donato, "Scienza e teologia nelle congregazioni romane: La questione atomista, 1626-1727," in Antonella Romano, ed., *Rome et la science moderne: Entre Renaissance et Lumières* (Rome, 2008), 595-634. See also Susana Gomez Lopez, *Le passioni degli atomi Montanari e Rossetti: Una polemica tra galileiani* (Florence, 1997).

tion.[47] The balance in power and dominant orientation in the curia shifted. A watershed moment was reached with the condemnation of quietism in 1687 and the wave of repression that ensued. Soon afterwards, in August 1689, Innocent XI died. Within weeks, two powerful protectors of both quietism and natural philosophy, cardinal Azzolino and Queen Christina, also died, as did prince Colonna.[48] Cardinal Pietro Ottoboni, the leader of the intransigent faction, was elected Pope Alexander VIII.

It was in these circumstances that attacks on natural philosophers gained a foothold, blurring any distinction between Cartesians, Gassendists, non-Aristotelian critics of Descartes, Galileans, Spinozists (whom some in Rome regarded as a branch of Cartesians), and atomists both old and new.[49]

Suspicion fell on medical circles in Naples, Siena, Pisa and Brescia.[50] Physicians were the most obvious proponents of such novelties. In addition, they were laity and close to political power without being powerful themselves.[51]

---

47 Gianvittorio Signorotto, "The squadrone volante: 'Independent' Cardinals and European Politics in the Second Half of the Seventeenth Century," in Gianvittorio Signorotto and Maria Antonietta Visceglia, eds., *Court and Politics in Papal Rome, 1492-1700* (Cambridge, 2002), 177-211.

48 Because Molinism taught inner illumination and passivity, it implied disrespect for external piety, which was the core of Counter-Reformation Catholicism. Because Molinos taught that the illuminated soul cannot do anything wrong, sexual misconduct could be justified. Molinism could thus meet libertinism, and both could verge on, and draw from, plain anticlericalism. Notably, all the Bianchi were said to have criticised the Inquisition for the Molinos affair.

49 On the Inquisition's view of the link between Descartes and Spinoza and the condemnation of Spinoza's *Opera posthuma* precisely in August 1690, see Leen Spruit and Pina Totaro, "Introduction," in *The Vatican Manuscript of Spinoza's Ethics* (Leiden, 2011), 1-59.

50 Lucio Amabile, *Il Santo Officio della Inquisizione a Napoli* (Città di Castello, 1892), esp. 56-60; Luciano Osbat, *L'inquisizione a Napoli. Il processo agli ateisti 1688-1697* (Rome, 1974). For Siena, where the main suspect was Pirro M. Gabrielli, a professor of botany and theoretical medicine, see ACDF, *Decreta Sancti Officii*, 1690, f. 226r, and Chiara Crisciani *et al.*, eds., *Scienziati a Siena* (Siena, 1999). On Pisa, see Paolo Galluzzi, "La scienza davanti alla chiesa e al principe in una polemica universitaria del secondo Seicento," in Luigi Borgia *et al.*, eds., *Studi in onore di Arnaldo d'Addario* (Lecce, 1995), vol. 4, 1317-1344; Gomez, *Le passion*. For Brescia – where the inquisitor seized a booklet by Francesco Ferdinando Ragazzini, *La medicina posta all'esame del tribunale della verità*, which Rome eventually allowed – see ACDF, St. St. O1n, n° 13.

51 This is very clear in the case of Lionardo di Capua's *Parere sopra l'incertezza della medicina* (Naples, 1681), which was reported in 1693 for praising Democritus. See Marta Fattori, "Censura e filosofia moderna: Napoli, Roma e l'affaire di Capua," *Nouvelles de la République des lettres*, 17 (2004), 23-44. *Pyrologia topographica*, by Domenico Bottone (Naples, 1692), the Viceroy's physician, was also denounced; Roman censors did not prohibit the

Attacks on *novatores* combined science and politics, in the sense that the practitioners affected were usually close to reformist parties at court, and that reported suspect propositions featured criticism of the papacy and the Inquisition: being "men of free philosophy," as the British travellers described Italian virtuosi, invariably implied that they deplored the very existence of the Inquisition.[52]

In Rome, too, at the first signs of such a grave controversy, elite physicians became suspect, and the more so as the protection they enjoyed had evaporated with the end of Lancisi's tenure as papal physician and the death of the *Congresso medico*'s patrons, the cardinals Azzolino, Pio and Rospigliosi. In a world where, in the Inquisitors' eyes, enemies of the Church were everywhere, there was no longer place for either audacious speculation or impiety – physicians were dangerously close to both. In the new balance of power, they were the obvious target.

Thus, as soon as on August 16, 1690 the inquisitors decided to curb the activities of all these high-profile physicians. They asked cardinal Vicar Gaspare Carpegna to summon Brasavola, to show him the "orders already given by this Sacred Congregation," and to order him and his fellows to never again "argue and defend [the theory] that substantial composites [are made of] atoms, and admonish his fellows."[53]

Paradoxically, had the inquisitors taken the time to read the defendants' writings, they would also have found, amidst praise for Descartes, Gassendi and their followers, rebuttals of their ideas on generation, respiration and animal sensation, consistently with the conventions of learned *medicina practica* that drew eclectically upon ancient and modern authorities. But Roman inquisitors were not usually keen treating lay people with excessive caution (although, obviously, much depended on their status). Whereas the long Latin treatises authored by ecclesiastics were examined with care, a proclivity for abridgement was strong towards the laity: an admonishment did not require a formal judgment to be dispensed.

Subsequently, while pursuing the investigation against the Bianchi, inquisitors dealt with Lancisi. They summoned his barber, who confirmed that

---

book, yet asked Bottone to amend what they considered suspect in his atomistic meteorology, see ACDF, *Censurae librorum* 1690-1692, n° 3.

52   Thomas Burnett, *Letters* (Rotterdam, 1686), 187-191.

53   "Nec ipse nec alii audeant substinere, et defendere compositiones substantiales ex atomis, et quod suos conacademicos moneat, eique ostendat ordines alias datos super huiusmodi materia a Sacra Congretagatione Sancti Offitii": ACDF, St. St. L5f, f. 183r; *Decreta Sancti Officii*, 1690, f. 258r.

Lancisi had had an affair with Chiara, and that her motive was revenge. As I have indicated, they also heard Lancisi himself for a second time, and received his confession. Eventually, the cardinals decided not to take the matter further. In his case, because testimonies came from socially inferior and morally untrustworthy witnesses, and because he had ostensibly changed his lifestyle and environment in the meanwhile, they reckoned that an admonishment would suffice; likewise, an admonishment was given to *monsignor* Del Noce. Both men's files would be preserved in the archive to be consulted in case of a relapse. The Roman Inquisition's methods were sometimes as unspectacular as they were persuasive.

Concluding Remarks: Philosophy and the Art of Medicine

The Inquisition's activism did not lead to any formal general prohibition of modern physics that some had feared. Polemics on the orthodoxy of atomism continued for a while, then subsided.[54]

In Rome, too, things quietly settled (though the Bianchi were severely punished). The *Congresso medico* did not survive, but as early as in 1691, Brasavola and Sinibaldi applied for the post of physician to the conclave.[55] Brasavola resumed his office at the papal household under Innocent XII, and Sinibaldi progressed at the university, at court and in the collegiate organisation. Gerosi became the Holy Office's physician.[56]

As for Lancisi, he achieved everything a physician could aspire to. He became Pope Clement XI's physician and trusted adviser, Chair of practical medicine, and *protomedicus*. He served as an expert for the Congregation of Rites in canonisation proceedings, always keeping that moderately sceptical stance which he shared with reformist circles in the curia and Church. Yet he kept a relic of Innocent XI, whom he regarded as a saint.[57] In 1714, at the height of his career, he created a library at the Santo Spirito where prospective doctors and

---

54   Maurizio Torrini, *Dopo Galileo: Una polemica scientifica (1684-1711)* (Florence, 1979); Vincenzo Ferrone, *Scienza natura religione: Mondo newtoniano e cultura italiana nel primo Settecento* (Naples, 1992); Donato, *Scienza*; Gustavo Costa, *Epicreismo e pederastia: Il "Lucrezio" e l'"Anacreonte" di Alessandro Marchetti secondo il Sant'Uffizio* (Florence, 2012).

55   ACDF, St. St. UV35, unnumbered ff.

56   ACDF, *Privilegi S. Officii Urbis 1669-1699*, f. 702r. I thank Bradford Bouley for this document.

57   Bradford A. Bouley, *Pious Postmortems: Anatomy, Sanctity, and the Catholic Church in Early Modern Europe* (Philadelphia, PA, 2017), 82. Lancisi gave his testimony in Pope Odescalchi beatification process, see *Romana Beatificationis et canonizationis Ven. Servi Dei Innocentii papae undecimi* (Rome, 1713), 6.

surgeons could familiarise themselves with ancient and modern texts, including, of course, the prohibited works, which might, nonetheless, offer useful insights into the art of healing. In his last testament and will, Lancisi left a substantial donation for a women's ward.

One might regard these activities as a gauge of hypocrisy or, less anachronistically, positional adjustments. Coping with the Inquisition was part of the wider configuration of power in which physicians were embedded, and which sustained their social roles while delimiting them. Practitioners dealt with such complexities depending on their status, age, and allegiances. Lancisi, the papal physician, could afford to be one and the same person with the sceptic, the pious physician, the learned courtier and the mechanical philosopher, gaining respectability from all.

As regards medical ideas, nothing appears to have changed for the physicians involved in the 1690 trial, either. Both Sinibaldi and Lancisi continued to teach in the same terms as before, the former favouring a chemically modernised Galenism, the latter a mechanical view of the body.[58] The flexible format (ultimately based on Galen's *Art of Medicine*) allowed for the introduction of ancient and contemporary opinions without expressing any definitive preference for one or the other.

Yet a closer look at their writings, and at the medical output at the turn of the seventeenth and eighteenth century in general, reveals a shift in accent. Although not a novelty in itself, stronger emphasis was placed on the limited usefulness of debates on first principles for medicine – more precisely, the practice of medicine, the art of healing which ultimately was the very *raison d'être* of the medical profession in society.

Accordingly, in a dissertation of 1693, *Sul modo di filosofar nell'arte medica*, Lancisi defended the usefulness of anatomy and chemistry for the understanding of the body, arguing that, like the whole universe, the body is created in "weight, numbers and measure" and is "but an organic aggregate of fluids of different movement and solids of various forms." Nonetheless, he recommended avoiding "scholastic physics transmitted in the metaphysical way, as well as the insensible atoms of Epicurus and Democritus" and ideas of the "first particles and atoms, from which the human body has neither benefit nor harm." Only if the natural sciences are "brought into the art of medicine," they can lead it to perfection.[59]

---

58 Giacomo Sinibaldi, *Institutiones medicae practicae*, MS London, Wellcome Library 4613; Giovanni M. Lancisi, *Prolusiones et orationes variae*, MS Rome, BL, Lancisi 153, ff. 41r-44v, on glands, and ff. 45r-50v on subtle anatomy.

59 Published in *Galleria di Minerva*, 4/2, (1700), 33-37: "Rerum Opifex, ea quae creando in pondere numero et mensura per universam Orbis molem disperserat in uno micorcosmo

From the late 1690s onwards there are, to the best of my knowledge, no records of experimental attempts to prove the existence of atoms, at least in
Rome. Academies of natural philosophy died out. The existence of corpuscles
was taken for granted; authors no longer attempted to prove their existence,
but restricted themselves to their physical operations. The Inquisition ensured
that they did not reappear *ex cathedra*.[60]

Relinquishing speculation on the ultimate nature of corpuscles did not,
however, prevent Roman and Italian physicians from developing interpretations of the body that were solely based upon material principles; this did not
exclude the possibility that matter could be endowed with intrinsic properties
other than shape and size, depending on the scale of observation. Once lip
service had been paid to Catholic dogma on the immortal rational soul, and
once problematic notions such as matter and form had been avoided, anything
else could be explored within the scope of practical medicine, including the
mind-body problem, framed in dualistic terms. The eclectic use of notions
such as corpuscles, mechanism and machine, by authors like Lorenzo Bellini,
Malpighi, Lancisi, Giorgio Baglivi, Domenico Gagliardi and Alessandro Pascoli,
finds its justification in the stated ultimate aim of medicine, that is, the main-
tainance or recovery of health – which only learned physicians were able to
perform. A mechanical view of life itself was purported in Rome by authors
like Lancisi and Baglivi, who, however, took care to frame it within the context
of practical medicine.[61] Anatomy and morbid anatomy, which already enjoyed
a strong tradition in Italy, became established as the specific empirical basis
for medical knowledge; the anatomical method, in turn, enhanced mechanism

---

mirabiliter coniunxerit. Siquidem Humanum corpus nilaliud est quam organicum aggre-
gatum ex fluidis etherogeneis diversimode motis, nec non ex solidis diversimodo figura-
tis"; "non ad scholasticam sese conferant phisicam, metaphisico modo traditam [...] non
ad insensibilia Democriti atomorum principia"; "omissisprimis particulis, atque atomis,
unde nihil periculi nihil commodi est nostro corpori"; "postremo in arte medica laborem
collocet omnem."

60   In 1706, for instance, the professor of medicine at the University of Perugia, Lodovico
Martinelli, was admonished by the local inquisitor not to teach the "doctrine of atoms, so
dangerous for our holy Faith": ACDF, St. St. UV60, n° 20 and *Censurae librorum 1704-1705*,
n° 4.

61   Mirko D. Grmek, *La première revolution biologique: Réflexions sur la physiologie et la médecine du XVIIe siècle* (Paris, 1990); François Duchesneau, *Les modèles du vivant de Descartes
à Leibniz* (Paris, 1998); and Luigi Guerrini, *Il grande affare della sapienza umana: Scienza e
filosofia nell'opera di Alessandro Pascoli (1669-1757)* (Florence, 2000), who, however, disre-
gards the distinctively medical approach of these authors. Further on Malpighi's gnoseol-
ogy, see Domenico Bertoloni Meli, ed., *Marcello Malpighi Anatomist and Physician*
(Florence, 1997).

in that it put some emphasis on the solid parts of the body and their healthy and diseased structures.[62]

A clear example of the negotiation between the old and the new, empiricism and tradition, expertise and authority, is Lancisi's first major work, *De subitaneis mortibus*. Lancisi describes the rational soul as "commanding" and "moving" the body only once, and then treats the body and life itself as the "non-hindered power of the animal machine to move the fluids of major function," and more precisely the "constant flow and reflow [...] of air, blood, [and] nerve juice through and from the organs of major function [which must be] in sufficiently good state," based on evidence from autopsies.[63] However, *De subitaneis mortibus* is essentially meant to teach physicians how to act when someone is struck by a sudden ailment, and how to prevent this by using the right treatment and regimen – eventually restating Galen's advice on how to live a healthy, regulated and ultimately pious life, under the physician's guidance.[64]

To conclude: Elena Brambilla once noted that, due to inquisitorial control, eighteenth-century Italian medicine did not engage in contemporary scientific developments, favouring an eclectic conciliation between the ancients and the moderns.[65] Here it is argued that such an assessment should be the starting point for exploring the ways in which physicians addressed philosophical issues precisely within practical medicine. If the ecclesiastical injunction to refrain from metaphysics was influential in shaping Italian medicine, this should be further investigated, taking into account how medical, philosophical and religious considerations were recast both in medical theory and practice, as well as in the professional ideology that underpinned the physician's role in society.

---

62   W.F. Bynum, "The Anatomical Method, Natural Theology, and the Functions of the Brain," *Isis*, 64 (1973), 444-468; Charles T. Wolfe, ed., *Medical Vitalism in the Enlightenment*, themed issue of *Science in Context,* 21/4 (2008); Maria Pia Donato, "Il normale, il patologico e la sezione cadaverica in età moderna," *Quaderni storici,* 46 (2011), 75-98; more in general, Matthew Landers and Brian Muñoz, eds., *Anatomy and the Organization of Knowledge, 1500-1850* (London, 2012).

63   Giovanni M. Lancisi, *De subitaneis mortibus* (Rome, 1707), in his *Opera,* 2: "vita est potentia, non impedita, machinae animalium ad motum fluidorum majoris usus"; "continuus, praeside ac movente anima, fluxus, ac refluxus plus minusve sensibilis aeris, sanguinis et liquidi nervorum per organa, et ex organis majoris usus, satis probe constitutis, et mutuo, atque alterne plus minusve sensibiliter agitatis et agitantibus."

64   Maria Pia Donato, *Sudden Death: Medicine and Religion in 18th-Century Rome* (Farnham, 2014).

65   Brambilla, "La medicina."

Contra medicos: Physicians Facing the Inquisition in Sixteenth-Century Venice

Alessandra Celati
Stanford University/University of Verona
alessandra.celati83@gmail.com; acelati@stanford.edu

Abstract

Since the Middle Ages, ecclesiastical authorities considered medical activity worthy of their attention and control. During the Counter-Reformation, they toughened their disciplinary action, aware of the peculiarity of an *ars* that mixed together the cure of the body with the cure of the soul. Moreover, the authorities became increasingly suspicious of practitioners who were highly involved in the Reformation movement, and who distanced themselves from Catholicism in the epistemological premises of their work. By examining original sources from the Venetian Inquisition archive, this paper discusses the factors that put the Roman Church and the medical profession in opposition to each other in the sixteenth century, and describes the professional solidarity put forward by physicians. It also examines the problematic relationship between doctors and the Inquisition, dealing with the former as effective agents of heretical propaganda.

Keywords

Inquisition – Venice – Protestant Reformation – physicians

The Venetian Inquisition has long attracted the interest of historians and historians of medicine due to the numerous areas at the intersection of medicine, culture and religion in the early modern Republic of Venice. The extremely rich Inquisition archives, now held in Venice's *Archivio di Stato* and in other provincial sites in the former Republic, have proven invaluable in addressing topics such as witchcraft, pretense of holiness, natural magic, possession and

---

* Dipartimento di Culture e Civiltà, Viale dell'Università 4, 37129, Verona, Italy.

mental illness, and popular healing practices.[1] Some scholars have also recently investigated the role of medical doctors in the repressive apparatus of the Inquisition.[2] Outstanding figures from the medical world whose works were prohibited have also been dealt with in detail.[3] However, although the spread of evangelism and Lutheranism *per se* has been the object of a vast body of scholarship, the reception of Protestantism in medical circles, and the related reaction of the Inquisition, has only been dealt with once.[4] In an article titled "Physicians and the Inquisition in Sixteenth-Century Venice," Richard Palmer describes the problematic relationship between physicians and the Holy Office, focussing in particular on one relevant case study, that of Girolamo Donzellini (of whom I, too, will speak in the following pages).[5]

In this paper, I widen the scope of the inquiry to the whole territory of the Republic. Grounded in a systematic analysis of original Inquisition archive sources, I will trace the medical doctors investigated by the *Savi all'Eresia* in the period between 1540 and 1575. This examination will allow me to take into account the peculiarity of the medical profession in its relationship with religious non-conformity, from an epistemological, methodological and social point of view. I argue that, although Venice's ecclesiastical authorities were most worried by the alleged faithlessness of medical *milieux*, the spread of reformed ideas in the medical environment was more than a sociological phenomenon in an age of general spiritual turmoil.[6] Indeed, there was a deeper intellectual connection between medicine and religious dissent. Medical practitioners were additionally targeted by the Inquisition because of their heretical propaganda activity. Practicing with different types of people, being

---

1 Ruth Martin, *Witchcraft and the Inquisition in Venice, 1550-1650* (Oxford, 1989); Jonathan Seize, *Witchcraft and Inquisition in Early Modern Venice* (Cambridge, 2011); Anne Jacobson Schutte, *Aspiring Saints: Pretence of Holiness, Inquisition, and Gender in the Republic of Venice, 1618-1750* (Baltimore, MD, and London, 2001); Sabina Minuzzi, *Sul filo dei segreti: Farmacopea, libri e pratiche terapeutiche a Venezia in età moderna* (Milan, 2016).

2 Federico Barbierato, "Il medico e l'inquisitore: Note su medici e perizie mediche nel tribunale del Sant'Uffizio veneziano fra Sei e Settecento," in Alessandro Pastore and Giovanni Rossi, eds., *Paolo Zacchia, alle origini della medicina legale: 1584-1659* (Milan, 2008), 266-285.

3 Ugo Baldini and Leen Spruit, *Catholic Church and Modern Science: Documents from the Archives of the Roman Congregations of the Holy Office and the Index*, vol. 1: *The Sixteenth Century* (Rome, 2009).

4 On the Reformation movement in Venice see John Martin, *Venice's Hidden Enemies: Italian Heretics in a Renaissance City* (Berkeley, CA, 1993); Paul F. Grendler, *The Roman Inquisition and the Venetian Press, 1540-1605* (Princeton, NJ, 1975).

5 Richard Palmer, "Physicians and the Inquisition in Sixteenth-Century Venice: The Case of Girolamo Donzellini," in Ole Peter Grell and Andrew Cunningham, eds., *Medicine and the Reformation* (London and New York, NY, 1993), 118-133.

6 See Maria Pia Donato's article in this volume.

well respected because of their specific professional mission (unless they pursued the accumulation of money more than the patients' health), and as men of culture accustomed to sophisticated philosophical discussions, they could propagate heretical beliefs from a privileged social position.

Medicine and the Inquisition in Sixteenth-Century Venice

In the sixteenth century Venice was notoriously "the gateway of the Reformation" in Italy.[7] It was one of the most prosperous Christian cities, a cosmopolitan town welcoming immigrants from all over Europe, and a highly developed centre of printing. The University of Padua – at the time probably the most renowned for the study of medicine and philosophy in Italy and abroad – also contributed to making the Republic a dynamic centre for cultural, philosophical and theological debates. Because the *Serenissima* was a fierce opponent of Roman political and jurisdictional claims, Venetian authorities created an autonomous Inquisitorial tribunal, the *Savi all'Eresia*, in which laymen worked side by side with clergymen, trying to mitigate the strength of the Roman action within the Venetian territory. This, in turn, supported the reputation of the *Serenissima* as a tolerant place.

The Republic, therefore, appealed to those interested in religious experimentation. Especially in Venice, there was a wide circulation of books by Protestant authors, and doctrinal discussions were held in the streets, the houses, the bookshops and the apothecaries. Among men of culture interested in the theological debate, physicians were numerous, and they often held leading positions in the Venetian heretical circles. It should, therefore, not come as a surprise that the medical profession caught the eye of the Inquisition.

In the second half of the sixteenth century, while the repression of heresy increased throughout Italy, the entire medical profession was put under the control of the Holy Office. Theoretically, all physicians had long been subject to the rules imposed by the ecclesiastical hierarchy. In particular, they had to fulfil the most basic rule, the canon issued in 1215 by Pope Innocent III, which required patients to confess their sins in order to be cured. Yet, in 1558, when the patriarch of Venice summoned the *priore* of the city's College of Physicians and asked him to request of all physicians that they abandon any patients who did not confess after the second medical visit, the College, firmly and unanimously, replied that physicians could not be forced to impose such a thing.[8] This was the beginning of a long fight. A file in the Venice Inquisition archive

---

7   See the letter that Bernardino Ochino wrote on December 7, 1542, quoted in Massimo Firpo, *Riforma protestante ed eresie nell'Italia del '500: Un profilo storico* (Rome and Bari, 1993), 17.

8   Venice, Biblioteca Marciana, MS Ital VII (2342=9695), *Notizie cavate dai libri dei priori*, f. 9v.

titled *"Contra medicos"* documents how the tensions between the physicians and the Holy Office increased in the course of the century.[9]

Since antiquity illness had been described as caused by both natural and moral causes. As a result, medical care was inherently suspended between a physical and a spiritual dimension and, over the course of the centuries, physicians were increasingly put under the control of ecclesiastical institutions.[10] In the second half of the sixteenth century, while the repression of heresy increased throughout Italy, Pious V issued the papal bull *Super gregem dominicum* (1566), which aggravated the regulations already contained in the 1215 *decretale*. The bull established that any doctor breaking the rule concerning the confession of patients would be expelled from the College of Physicians, deprived of the academic qualification of 'doctor in medicine and philosophy,' and fined.[11] What is more, such violation entailed that the guilty physician was listed among those in the city suspected of heresy.[12]

---

9 Archivio di Stato di Venezia (hereafter ASV), Sant'Uffizio, *Processi: Contra medicos*, Busta (hereafter B.) 35. The episode is also examined in Palmer, "Physicians and the Inquisition," 120-121, and Alessandra Celati, "A Peculiar Reformed Minority: Italian Protestant Physicians between Religious Propaganda, Inquisition Repression and Freedom of Thought," forthcoming in Simon Burton, Michal Choptiany and Piotr Wilczec, eds., *Reformed Majorities and Minorities, Confessional Boundaries and Contested Identities* (Göttingen, 2018).

10 This link has been broadly analysed in historiography. See in particular: Vivian Nutton, "God, Galen and the Depaganization of Ancient Medicine," in Peter Biller and Joseph Ziegler, eds., *Medicine and Religion in the Middle Ages* (York, 2001), 17-32; Jole Agrimi and Chiara Crisciani, "Carità e assistenza nella civiltà cristiana medievale," in Mirko Grmek, ed., *Storia del pensiero medico occidentale*, vol. 1: *Antichità e medioevo* (Bari, 1993), 217-259; Joseph Ziegler, *Medicine and Religion, c. 1300: The Case of Arnau de Vilanova* (Oxford, 1998); John Henderson, *The Renaissance Hospital: Healing the Body and Healing the Soul* (New Haven, 2006); Maria Pia Donato, Luc Berlivet, *et al.*, eds., *Médecine et religion: Compétitions, collaborations, conflits (xiie-xxe siècles)* (Rome, 2013).

11 ASV, Sant'Uffizio, *Processi: Contra medicos*, B. 35. On the *Super Gregem Dominicum* Bull, the role of confession in the ecclesiastic authorities' strategy against the spread of heresy and the involvement of physicians in the Counter-Reformation see Alessandro Pastore, *Le regole dei corpi: Medicina e disciplina nell'Italia moderna* (Bologna, 2006), 136-137. On the implementation of the *Super Gregem Dominicum* papal bull in some Italian cities see Rosario Romeo, *Ricerche su confessione dei peccati e Inquisizione nell'Italia del Cinquecento* (Reggio Calabria, 1997), 107-114. The medical debate on the obligation to grant confession to the dying patient was continued between the seventeenth and the nineteenth century, see Maria Pia Donato, *Sudden Death: Medicine and Religion in Eighteenth-Century Rome* (Farnham, 2014), 162-165. In the same book the author also shows the extent to which death, especially if sudden, became a disciplining instrument in the hands of the post-Tridentine Catholic Church.

12 Charles Cocquelines, *Bullarum, privilegiorum ac diplomatum Romanorum Pontificum amplissima* (Rome, 1745), 281.

However, soon after the new regulation was issued, the College refused to apply it and stood against the Inquisition's demands to interfere in medical practice. This led to the most clamorous case of professional solidarity among Venetian physicians. On September 20, 1571, a parish priest named Antonio Rocha denounced all physicians in the city to the Inquisition, asserting that, "in their own interests," they had not made any efforts to convince their patients to confess and then receive the holy communion.[13] Rocha was referring to a specific episode that had recently taken place in his parish, but which was clearly not exceptional. A member of the College, Antonio Secco, allegedly did not invite his patient to confess, and, what was worse, when the patient himself asked to see the priest, Secco had replied that this was not necessary. As a consequence, the *gentil'uomo* died without having received the sacrament, which caused Rocha to file a complaint to the Inquisitors. The judges acknowledged that the episode was serious, and quickly summoned Aloisio Bagnolo, the *priore* of the College, in order to remind him of his religious duties and insist that he order his colleagues to respect the bull. Soon afterwards, the Holy Office published an official document which established that every breach of the bull (committed by whoever was in charge of patients' health, whether a collegiate physician or not) was to be interpreted as an act of rebellion and heresy, and was to be punished with a ban from practicing medicine and banishment from Venice.[14] At the same time, an inquisitorial decree was distributed all over the city by parish priests, announcing that, if sick, citizens had to call the confessor; if they did not, their physicians would be compelled to abandon them.

Such strong action by the Inquisition forced the *priore* to obey: reluctantly Aloisio Bagnolo summoned his colleagues and asked them to respect the bull (however, Antonio Secco was not prosecuted by the Inquisition in any way). However, the Inquisition did not obtain the expected result. The file *Contra medicos* shows that as early as in May 1572, that is, eight months after that the entire profession had been denounced to the Inquisitors, one member of the College, Prospero da Foligno, did not apply the Roman rules, which led to his patient dying without confession. He was denounced by the priest of the San

---

13   "Jo son venuto per discargar la coscientia [...] perche mi par una cosa mal fatta che li medici sotto pretesto di non voler gli infermi, o per qualche altro suo particolare interesse non si cureno di persuader li infermi a dover confessarsi et comunicarsi si come è intervenuto nella parocchia mia." ASV, Sant'Uffizio, *Processi: Contra medicos*, B. 35, denunciation dated September 20, 1571. See also Palmer, "Physicians and the Inquisition," 120-121.

14   ASV, Sant'Uffizio, *Processi: Contra medicos*, B. 35, inquisitorial decree dated October 16, 1571.

Zuan Grisostomo parish and was promptly summoned by the Inquisition in order to be interrogated. When Prospero was asked about the reason for his negligence he failed to adduce any convincing argument, and merely replied: "I have no answer for this."[15] The source is incomplete, so we cannot know what happened to Prospero, who was summoned for a second interrogatory in the following week, which is, however, not recorded in the file. Nevertheless, we do know that he attended the College's meeting until 1575: enjoying his colleagues' protection, he was able to get away with his breach of the Roman rules.

Indeed, while the Inquisition insisted on trying to make physicians bend to its will, the physicians kept attempting to evade ecclesiastical control. In 1579 and in 1589 the *priore* was summoned again, and again he was asked to make his colleagues respect the papal bull, which is an indication that, in their ordinary practice, medical doctors did not observe the Roman injunctions. In fact, on both occasions, speaking on behalf of the entire profession, the *priore* stated that applying the *Super Gregem Dominicum* was "not doable" because of "many difficulties."[16]

The Venetian physicians' reaction to the interference of the Church was somewhat peculiar in mid-16th-century Italy. At that time, most Colleges of Physicians included in their statutes the rule that imposed patient confessions, and approved repressive measures against heretical physicians, in order to please the Roman Church and thereby strengthen the honour of the profession.[17]

It is worth comparing the Venetian College of Physicians with doctors' professional resistance to ecclesiastical intrusion elsewhere. In Modena, for instance, reformed doctrines had been spreading since the 1530s, and the medical community played an important role in the local heretical movement.[18] For

---

15   "Io non vi so rispondere di questo," ibid.

16   Venice, Biblioteca Marciana, MS Ital VII (2342=9695), *Notizie cavate dai libri dei priori*, f. 17v. In 1579 "i 4 savi ordine (sic) dell'inquisizione al collegio che li medici non visitino li infermi che non si confessano. Risposta del collegio non potervisi questo eseguire per cinque ragioni." Ten years later the *priore* was summoned again "perché faci osservare da medici la bulla di Pio V circa il visitar chi non si confessa. Risulse il collegio rispondere et addir le difficoltà," ibid, f. 21r.

17   On the acceptance of the Roman Church's pressures on controlling medical practice see in particular the case of the College of Physicians in Verona, and the one of the College of Physicians in Cremona: Alessandro Pastore, "L'onore della corporazione: Il Collegio medico di Verona tra il tardo Quattrocento e gli inizi del Seicento," in Maurizio Zangarini, ed., *Studi di storia per Luigi Ambrosoli* (Verona, 1993), 7-28; Luigi Belloni, "Gli statuti del Collegio dei Fisici di Cremona," *Bollettino storico cremonese* (1995-1997), 5-46.

18   On the spread of heresy in Modena see: Massimo Firpo, "Gli 'spirituali,' l'Accademia di

this reason, in 1550, the local College of Physicians approved new regulations, intended to safeguard therapeutic activity from the Inquisition's control. More precisely, it established that the College meetings were secret, and that physicians were not compelled to fulfil the city's laws if these contrasted with their deontological duty. The statutes bore no reference to Innocent III's *decretale*, which was obviously dangerous for practitioners favouring heresy. The reform of the statutes was actually approved a few months after Pope Julius III had issued a decree which assured mercy to every heretic who 'spontaneously' surrendered and denounced his accomplices. This decree also established that, in case of a suspicion of heterodoxy, the confessor could impose the *spontanea comparizione*, under the threat of an Inquisitorial trial.[19]

Domizia Weber has convincingly argued that Modenese physicians, who probably shared non-conformist religious ideas and books with their patients, now feared that their heretical tenets could be exposed, and tried to protect themselves by reducing their patients' opportunities to get in touch with confessors.[20] Bearing this in mind, we can suppose that in Modena, and even more so in Venice, where the Reformation movement had been strong and hence where physicians had played an important part in the spread of heresy, the medical profession as a whole opposed interferences from Rome in a particularly tenacious way. The Modenese College's statutes did not even include the rule in 1580, when the *Super Gregem Dominicum* was published in the city (the delay was due to the persisting refusal of bishop Morone to publish the bull as long as he was alive).[21] So, if it is possible to consider the bull a 'weapon' meant to eradicate once and for all the resistance of the medical profession, it is also arguable that, at least in some cities, this was an ineffective means. In Venice

Modena e il formulario di fede del 1542: Controllo del dissenso religioso e nicodemismo," in idem, *Inquisizione romana e controriforma: Studi sul cardinal Giovanni Morone e il suo processo d'eresia* (Bologna, 1992), 55-130; Susanna Peyronel Rambaldi, *Speranze e crisi nel Cinquecento Modenese: Tensioni religiose e vita cittadina ai tempi di Giovanni Morone* (Milan, 1997); Matteo Al Kalak, *L'eresia dei fratelli: Una comunità eterodossa nella Modena del Cinquecento* (Rome, 2011).

19   Elena Brambilla in Adriano Prosperi, ed., *Dizionario storico dell'Inquisizione*, vol. 3 (Pisa, 2010), s.v. "Spontanea comparizione (procedura sommaria)," 834-836.

20   Domizia Weber, *Sanare e maleficiare: Guaritrici, streghe e medicina a Modena nel XVI secolo* (Rome, 2011), 97-121.

21   See the letter that Giovanni Crepona sent to the Este Duke Alfonso II, on January 22, 1580, quoted in Weber, *Sanare e maleficiare*, 119. On Giovanni Morone see Massimo Firpo and Dario Marcatto, *Il processo inquisitoriale del Cardinal Giovanni Morone: Nuova edizione critica*, vols. 1-3 (Vatican City, 2011-2015).

and in Modena professional solidarity was stronger than reverence for the Church.

Speaking of professional solidarity, it is also worth mentioning that the *Savi all'Eresia* archives preserve evidence of physicians acting as witnesses in support of colleagues put on trial by the Inquisition – independently of how serious the allegations were. Antonio Secco (the same physician who was the protagonist in the *Contra medicos* affair) defended Decio Bellebuono when the latter was brought in front of the judges for heresy in 1567.[22] In the same year, the member of the College Lelio Rama informed his colleague Vincenzo Negroni that a trial was going to be set up against him.[23] Hercole Manzoni testified in 1588 in defence of Pier Paolo Malvezzi, who was accused of atheism and incest.[24] Clearly, the Venetian College rejected the Inquisition's claims of control on both ethical and deontological grounds, and because of the impressively high quantity of physicians involved in the city's heretical movement.

"The Best Physician Is also a Philosopher": Medicine and Heresy among Learned Physicians

The Venetian medical world was particularly receptive to Protestantism and other strands of religious dissent. A systematic survey of the Inquisition records, combined with the study of the sources related to the activity of the College of Physicians, allows one to calculate the percentage of non-conformist doctors in the city. Roughly 25% of the total number of those who practiced medicine in Venice between 1540 and 1575 were inclined towards reformed positions.[25]

---

22 ASV, Sant'Uffizio, *Processi: Ad defensam Antonii Volpe de Ferrandina*, B. 23, see the deposition Secco gave on July 11, 1567. On Decio Bellebuono see William Eamon, "The Canker Friar: Piety and Intrigue in an Era of New Diseases," in Franco Mormando and Thomas Worcester, eds., *Piety and Plague: From Byzantium to the Baroque* (Kirksville, MO, 2007), 156-176.

23 ASV, Sant'Uffizio, *Processi: Contro Vincenzo Negroni*, B. 22, see the accused's interrogatory dated April 12, 1567.

24 ASV, Sant'Uffizio, *Processi: Contro Pier Paolo Malvezzi*, B. 46, see the deposition dated September 17, 1588.

25 The calculations on which this output is based are discussed in Alessandra Celati, *Medici ed eresie nel Cinquecento italiano* (PhD dissertation, University of Pisa, 2016), 306-313. For a statistical examination of all the trials set up in Venice against religious dissenters (most of whom generically defined as 'Lutherans'), see John Tedeschi and William Monter, "Toward a Statistical Profile of the Italian Inquisitions, Sixteenth to Eighteenth Centuries,"

The widespread circulation of reformed doctrines among medical doctors was due to many reasons, and in particular to the peculiar way physicians understood their professional role. The Italian heretical physician Girolamo Massari, who was compelled to flee from the Republic of Venice to Basel in 1551 for religious reasons, clearly maintained in his *Eusebius captivus*, a pamphlet against the Roman Inquisition, that, as a physician, it was his duty to deal with spiritual matters as well as with natural ones.[26] He explained the reasons why he decided to write about religious issues: "Not only does the physician need to know and to understand bodies, but he also has to show what the true medicine for souls is." Quoting Galen, he added that: "Since the good physician has to be an excellent philosopher, he is not forbidden from dealing with the aim of philosophy, that is to say: looking for the truth of things."[27] And finally, as though medicine and religion were one, Massari concluded:

> As a matter of fact, the writing of the holy history of the deeds of the Apostles did not cloud Luke's medical profession, and it actually showed that the man who was able to administer remedies to the bodies could reveal the celestial medicine to the souls as well.[28]

The overlap between curing the body and curing the soul, and the references to Luke the Evangelist, who was the patron of physicians, were commonplace in sixteenth-century medical culture. Following Galen's teachings, some sixteenth-century *medici-philosophi* actually thought that philosophy *was* the medicine of the soul, which possibly inspired a peculiar sense of their professional mission. It legitimated a claim to deal with sacred matters which, in

---

      now in John Tedeschi, *The Prosecution of Heresy: Collected Studies on the Inquisition in Early Modern Italy* (Binghamton, NY, 1991), 105.

26   On Girolamo Massari see Achille Olivieri in *Dizionario biografico degli Italiani*, vol. 71 (Rome, 2008), s.v. "Girolamo Massari", 359-380; Michaela Valente, *Contro l'Inquisizione: Il dibattito europeo (XVI-XVIII secolo)* (Turin, 2009), 34-46.

27   See the well-known work by Galen: *Quod optimus medicus sit quoque philosophus*.

28   Girolamo Massari, *Eusebius captivus, sive modus procedendi in curia romana contra luteranos, in quo praecipua Christianae religionis capita examinantur: Trium dierum actis absolutus* (Basel, 1553), 18. "Quanquam ne corporis quidem humani medicum dedecere arbitror, ut agnoscat, unamque ostendat, quae vera animorum sit medicina. Medico namque qui etiam optimus philosophus sit oportet, ut inquit Galenus, philosophiae scopum, qui ipsa est veritas rerum, ac morum probitas, pertractare non denegandum est. Neque enim Lucae medicam professionem obscuravit historiae sanctissimae de gestis Apostolorum scriptio, sed potius illustravit, ut qui corporibus medelam afferre noverat, idem quoque animis coelestem indicaret."

turn, could result in a rational approach to theology: it was a short step from there to the adherence to non-conformist positions.

Massari's *Eusebius captivus* is not the only textual evidence for this. A polemicist hidden behind the name of Alphonsus Lyncurius Terraconensis referred to the example of Saint Luke in order to defend and eulogize Miguel Servetus, the well-known Spanish physician and theologian who was sentenced to death by Calvin in 1553. According to Lyncurius, Servetus' shift from medical to theological inquiry, with the purpose of revealing the true essence of Christianity, deserved special praise, as it mirrored the activity of the apostle.[29]

Servetus's case is particularly illuminating for the intersections between medicine and religion. As is well known, his thought combined theology, neo-platonic philosophy and anatomical research. In his quest to show how the Holy Spirit was inhaled by men he managed to discover pulmonary circulation.[30] Servetus' heresy lay in his divinization of man and in his denial of the doctrine of the Trinity. In fact, the three elements of the Trinity were nothing but different 'dispositions' of the singular God who pervaded the entire universe – as was taught by neo-platonic philosophy – and vivified man's soul through breath and the circulation of blood. Sharing Servetus' cultural background, considering themselves philosophers and interested in speculation that experimented with both medicine and theology, Italian physicians were naturally inclined to accept such positions. Indeed, historical sources show that Servetus' ideas, condemned by the Roman Inquisition as much as by Protestant churches, were circulated in oral form and that his books, *De trinitatis erroribus* and *Christianismi restitutio*, reached other cities in Italy precisely from Padua.[31] Even after Servetus was burnt at the stake in Geneva, his work

---

29   "Michael Servetus Villanovanus Tarraconensis, medicae artis peritissimus, Lucam illum medicum, cuius plurima in evangelio laus est, imitatus, quum plurimum ingenio valeret, et de veritate religionis mundum tumultuari nec non plurimorum scriptis et voluminibus infarciri satis aegre conspiceret, animum suum ad sacras literas subinde transtulit, in eisque omne suum Studium et ingenium collocavit." *Alphonsi Lyncurii terraconensis, Apologia pro M. Serveto*, in John Calvin, *Opera quae supersunt omnia*, vol. 15 (Brunswick, 1863-1900), 53. Traditionally, historiography identified Lyncurius with the Italian exiles Matteo Gribaldi or Celio Secondo Curione. According to Ángel Alcalá, nonetheless, it is not possible to rule out that behind the pseudonym was an unidentified Spanish Antitrinitarian, see Ángel Alcalá, ed., *Miguel Servet: Obras completas*, 6 vols (Saragozza, 2003), vol. 1, 287.

30   On Servet see Roland Bainton, *Hunted Heretic: The Life and Death of Michael Servetus, 1511-1553* (Boston, MA, 1960); Claudio Manzoni, *Umanesimo ed eresia: Michele Serveto* (Naples, 1974); Ángel Alcalá, ed., *Miguel Servet.*

31   Aldo Stella, *Anabattismo e antitrinitarismo in Italia nel XVI secolo* (Padua, 1969); Giuseppe

circulated in northern Italy, thanks to some professors at Padua university and physicians who worked in Veneto.[32]

Though the link between medicine and heterodoxy had epistemological grounds, it was also rooted in the vibrant cultural environment which physicians were breathing in during their study (especially, but not exclusively, those who graduated in Padua). Not only could they get in touch with dangerous doctrines, such as that of Servetus (not to mention the spread of Averroism), but the very philological method they became familiar with had an impact on their religious attitudes.[33]

Agostino Gadaldino, a physician from Modena who moved to Venice in the late 1530s or early 1540s is a case in point.[34] When he presented himself before the Inquisition in Venice in 1557 (taking advantage of the above-mentioned edict of grace issued by Julius III), he claimed that, as a man of culture, he was a curious person and, as such, he did not expect that "questioning the faith [in the Roman Church] was heretical."[35] His whole deposition is grounded in the legitimacy of "reasoning" on, and "questioning," Roman doctrines, while he never admitted to have outwardly embraced reformed tenets – actually holding positions that diverged enough from some of Protestants' key doctrinal points. He questioned the Pope's authority, the necessity of praying to the saints, the real presence of the body of Christ in the Eucharist, and the feasibility of the vow of chastity, but he continued to believe in the authority of the Councils, and he accepted confession as a sacrament. Of course, while on trial, Gadaldino would belittle his crimes, and he would refer instrumentally to his profession in order to justify his involvement with the heretical movement. Still, the *topos* of the man of culture interested in the religious debate because of his mental *habitus* cannot have been mere rhetoric. All physicians were familiar with books and were used to critical-philological textual analysis, but a

Ongaro, "La scoperta della circolazione polmonare e la diffusione della *Christianismi restitutio* di Michele Serveto nel XVI secolo in Italia e nel Veneto," *Episteme*, 5 (1971), 3-44.

32   Thanks to a letter written in 1560 by the Calvinist physician Guglielmo Gratarolo we find out that Servet's books (for instance *De trinitatis erroribus*) were smuggled to northern Italy (from Pietro Perna's printing house in Basel) from the 1550s onwards, especially through the agency of the Padua professor Matteo Gribaldi (but the above-mentioned Girolamo Massari was involved as well); see Leandro Perini, "Note e documenti su Pietro Perna libraio-tipografo a Basilea," *Nuova rivista storica*, 50 (1966), 162.

33   Martin Pine, *Pomponazzi Radical Philosopher of the Renaissance* (Rome and Padua, 1986).

34   Historians have never dealt in detail with this physician. For some information on him see the entry in the Italian biographical dictionary on his father: Alessandro Pastore in *Dizionario biografico degli Italiani*, vol. 51 (1998), s.v. "Gadaldino, Antonio", 128-131.

35   ASV, Sant'Uffizio, *Processi: Contro Agostino Gadaldino*, B. 13, August 3, 1557.

man like Gadaldino all the more so. Agostino was the son of a Modenese book-seller, who was well-known for his reformed positions. Growing up while attending to a bookshop filled with heretical works, Agostino had become familiar with heterodox readings. Even more important still, in 1541 he was in charge, as the chief editor, of the publication of Galen's *Opera omnia*.[36] He was supposed to check the philological accuracy of the texts and the precision of the translation from the Greek, and he devoted himself to this enterprise to such an extent that he eventually fell ill.[37]

The case of Gadaldino illustrates the extent to which, in the humanistic context, the new interest in reading the texts of the ancient authors in their original version stimulated a potentially heretical inquiry into Scripture, and also into ancient medical and philosophical works.[38] Thanks to their familiarity with ancient and modern texts, and to their philologically oriented learning methods, some humanist physicians were, arguably, receptive to a *sola scriptura* approach to religion. Moreover, in sharing a critical attitude towards knowledge, they were inclined to question religious dogmas and scholastic truths, while their very religious experience seems to have been the result of a rational, free-thinking, 'doubtful' approach to the sacred.

One might well object and observe that physicians shared a humanistic background and a critical-philological attitude with other professions, such as lawyers, who were, indeed, equally numerous in the Italian heretical movement. Nonetheless, medicine was in a peculiar position due to the epistemological shift it underwent in Italian universities in the course of the sixteenth century. At that time, medicine was increasingly being conceived as a pragmatic discipline, dealing with an inherently uncertain and unstable object: the individual human body and its illnesses. New emphasis was put both on the value of *conjecture* and on *practica rationale*.[39] This shift made an experiential approach possible, while avoiding a reduction of learned medicine to the em-

---

36   Stefania Fortuna, "The Latin Editions of Galen's *Opera omnia* (1490-1625) and Their Prefaces," *Early Science and Medicine*, 17 (2012), 391-412.

37   Charles Donald O'Malley, *Andreas Vesalius of Brussels, 1514-1564* (Berkeley, CA, 1964), 102-104.

38   On physicians' academic education, see Paul F. Grendler, *The Universities of the Italian Renaissance* (Baltimore, MD, 2002). On the heretical potential inherent even in the speculation of Catholic humanist physicians, see Jean-Michel Agasse, "Girolamo Mercuriale: Humanism and Physical Culture in the Renaissance," in Concetta Pennuto, ed., *Girolamo Mercuriale, De arte gymnastica* (Florence, 2008), 861-1110.

39   Simone Mammola, *La ragione e l'incertezza: Filosofia e medicina nella prima età moderna* (Milan, 2012).

pirical methods of quacks. Arguably, such an epistemological transformation changed the mind frame of sixteenth-century Italian physicians. A gradual move from tradition towards a more personal, independent search for new theories and solutions was made possible.

In other words, the epistemological and methodological framework of Renaissance medicine made it easily compatible with the Reformation. What is left to examine is the heretical physician's social role in the sixteenth-century Venetian context, and its significance with respect to the Inquisition's persecution of medical doctors.

Salus and Heretical Propaganda: A Few Cases

The medical practice put physicians in a peculiar social position, as they were able to develop an extensive network of relations with individuals from all social groups. This circumstance, along with their cultural dynamism and the contacts they had with colleagues, humanists and printers all over Italy and abroad, put physicians at the core of the heretical web. More specifically, patient and doctor developed an intimate relationship at the sickbed, which included, according to the Hippocratic-Galenic precepts, the discussion of the past, habits and spiritual life of the patient. To provide a contrast to pain and sickness, the physician was supposed to talk with his patient and help him recover emotional and physical balance. Medical doctors were supposed to prescribe a correct regimen, giving advice on food as well as on sexual habits, suggesting how much to move, sleep and work, and describing the physiological consequences of different emotional states. In so doing, physicians became 'global counsellors' for their patients. Following Galen, "the doctor believed that his treatment would be more effective if he had the trust of the patient."[40] The physician aimed to become "the faithful companion of the body of his patient": as part of his deontology, and as a necessary condition for the cure, he had to strike up a relation of empathy with the ill.[41] The relation which saw, on the one hand, men of culture, prone to philosophical discussion and theological debate, and, on the other hand, people weakened by illness, sometimes

---

40   Roger French, *Medicine Before Science: The Business of Medicine from the Middle Ages to the Enlightenment* (Cambridge, 2003), 146; Sandra Cavallo and Tessa Storey, *Healthy Living in Late Renaissance Italy* (Oxford, 2013).

41   Roger French, "The Medical Ethics of Gabriele de Zerbi," in Andrew Wear, Johanna Geyer-Kordesch and Roger French, eds., *Doctors and Ethics: The Earlier Historical Setting of Medical Ethics* (Amsterdam, 1993), 84.

socially and intellectually inferior, could lead the way to a pervasive propaganda developing in mutual protection and complicity.

Inquisitors were well aware of the religious potential of medical practice. When in 1571 an aristocrat from Pordenone, Alessandro Mantica, was put on trial for holding radical ideas, the judges asked him to prove that he had respected the *Super Gregem Dominicum* rules during the long illness from which he had suffered in 1566.[42] Moreover, they repeatedly tried to obtain information about the physician who had cured him – an unnamed medical doctor from Udine. One year previously, during the interrogation of Niccolò da Pavia, a heretic who had fled to Chiavenna before being caught by the Inquisition, the judges overtly asked whether any physician had helped him escape or had been an accomplice to his religious mistakes.[43]

In the *Savi all'Eresia* sources, there is sound evidence of Venetian physicians' attempt to carry out heterodox propaganda. For instance, Teofilo Panarelli, the leader of a Calvinist group in Venice, made fun of the relatives of a young patient of his, who wanted to call the priest in order to bless the girl. The physician laughed at this suggestion, asserting that this was a superstition and saying that: "People do so many things which offend God!"[44] What is more, shortly before being caught by the Inquisition, Panarelli assisted his comrade in faith and colleague Giuseppe Moscardo at the time of the latter's mortal illness, persuading him to stick to his Protestant beliefs and to refuse confession till the very end.[45]

Likewise, the medical doctor Girolamo Donzellini, who was repeatedly put on trial by the Holy Office, was able to convert two nuns in the convent of Santa Lucia while treating them.[46] He taught the two women heretical

---

42 ASV, Sant'Uffizio, *Processi: Contro Alessandro Mantica*, B. 34.

43 Mariano Mantese and Giovanni Nardello, *Due processi per eresia: La vicenda religiosa di Luigi Groto, il Cieco di Adria e della nobile vicentina Angelica Pigafetta-Piovene* (Vicenza, 1974), 99.

44 "Dicendo noi di casa di volerlo far segnare, questo medico cominciò a ridere e dir che queste erano superstizione, e soggionse: voi siete parenti a queste donnicciole che portano li bollettini e parole simili soggioggendo ancora in questo ragionamento: quante cose si fanno che sono contro l'honor di Dio." ASV, Sant'Uffizzio, *Processi: Contra Ludovico Abioso e Teofilo Panarelli*, B. 32; see the deposition that Grazioso Percacino gave on July 18, 1568. On Panarelli see Palmer, *Physicians and the Inquisition*, 121; Martin, *Venice's Hidden Enemies*, 159-160, 180-182.

45 ASV, Sant'Uffizio, *Processi: Contra Ludovico Abioso e Teofilo Panarelli*, B. 32; see Panarelli's interrogatory dated December 6, 1571. See also Palmer, "Physicians and the Inquisition," 121.

46 The figure of Girolamo Donzellini, a Venetian heretical doctor, has been examined in

doctrines and convinced them to break their vows and flee. Donzellini's case is well known to historians. Drawn into the reformed movement by his intellectual curiosity, he was open-minded enough to develop his own approach to religion (a spiritual, irenic, ethical version of Christianity). Being curious about the most innovative medical theories, such as those of Paracelsus and Fernel, he was able to combine them with traditional Galenism in an eclectic way; as an expert smuggler of prohibited texts and an insatiable reader, he was sentenced to death (after having survived four trials and one plague epidemic) for the possession of prohibited books.[47] Unsurprisingly, his heretical propaganda was pervasive and effective. In fact, Donzellini somewhat embodies the archetypical heretical medical doctor.

Although not as renowned as Donzellini's, the most significant case of religious propaganda by a Venetian medical doctor is probably that of Vincenzo Negroni, a collegiate physician put on trial in 1567.[48] Witnesses testified that for eight years Negroni had attended the holy Mass without making any effort to dissimulate his hostility toward Catholicism, and overtly mocking the preacher (whom he later tried to convert, too).[49] Negroni had been converted to Protestantism by a man named Pasqualino Boccalier; Pasqualino had assisted him during his illness, and "as a sign of gratitude for that service," Negroni became more and more involved in the Reformation movement.[50] As I pointed out above, the condition of being ill was in itself exploitable for the construction of heterodox relationships – even in cases when the sick person was himself a physician. In 1569 Negroni was sentenced to public recantation, something which was particularly humiliating for a man who made a living in a "profession nourished by honour."[51] The Inquisition's strategy was to mar-

---

Palmer, "Physicians and the Inquisition." On Donzellini, see further Anne Jacobson Schutte in *Dizionario biografico degli Italiani*, vol. 41 (Rome, 1992), s.v. "Donzellini, Girolamo", 238-243; Pastore, "L'onore della corporazione"; Alessandra Quaranta, *La rete di scambi epistolari fra medici italiani e di lingua tedesca nel XVI Secolo: Libertà di ricerca, circolazione del sapere ed esperienze confessionali*, (PhD dissertation, University of Trento, 2016). As far as original archive sources are concerned, see: ASV, Sant'Uffizio, *Processi: Contro Girolamo Donzellini*, B. 39.

47   Alessandra Celati, "Medicine, Heresy and Paracelsianism in Sixteenth-Century Italy: The Case of Girolamo Donzellini (1513-1587)," *Gesnerus*, 71 (2014), 5-37.

48   ASV, Sant'Uffizzio, *Processi: Contro Vincenzo Negroni medico*, B. 22.

49   ASV, Sant'Uffizzio, *Processi: Contro Vincenzo Negroni medico*, B. 22; see the deposition that one Antonio mercadante gave on March 22, 1567.

50   "Per rispetto della servitù che mi faceva nel tempo delle mie infermità," ASV, Sant'Uffizio, *Processi: Contro Vincenzo Negroni medico*, B. 22, interrogatory dated June 21, 1567.

51   I draw this expression ("ho fatto professione di mia arte che vive dell'onore") from the *apologia* that Girolamo Donzellini wrote for the judges in 1560, ASV, Sant'Uffizio, *Processi: Contro Girolamo Donzellini*, B. 39, f. 52r.

ginalise dissenting doctors and expulse them from any therapeutic context, if not physically eliminate them. As for Donzellini and Panarelli, they were sentenced to death despite their recantations.

The role of physicians as agents of heretical propaganda was even more successful outside the urban context. In small villages and in provincial towns, physicians enjoyed a relatively higher social status. This allowed them to take on the roles of cultural and social mediators, promoting complex theological doctrines by teaching them to the illiterates in a and comprehensible way. The doctor of medicine Antonio Massimo chose a *condotta* outside Venice with the declared intention of converting as many people as possible. As is reported in the denunciation, he thought that in the countryside the inquisitorial action was not as dangerous as it was in Venice. When he was living in the capital, Massimo had already habitually spoken overtly about his religious ideas and expressed them during his therapeutic activity. For instance, he lampooned the apparition of the Virgin Mary before a young patient of his, and scorned the patient's family's suggestion of making a vow to the *Madonna della Lanna* in order to help the girl recover.[52] However, according to the deposition the denouncer gave in 1560, Massimo was feeling disappointed about the results of the heretical activity he had been carrying out in Venice. He therefore decided to leave the city. First he moved to the area around Bergamo, and after a while he settled down in Oderzo, convinced that "this city was a softer ground [compared to Venice]."[53] Massimo had to reduce his hopes and ambitions over the course of the decade, until he totally abandoned them: in 1571 he was listed among the Italian religious exiles that had sought shelter in Geneva.[54]

In a rural context, amidst peasants and artisans, *medici condotti* (who did not share the high standards of their city colleagues) sometimes emphasised the social message of the Gospels in order to gain the trust and favour of the population.[55] Stefano de Giusti, an Anabaptist *medico condotto* who worked in Gardone, near Brescia, used to say that there was no point in making a difference between working and non-working days, especially for poor people who had to work in order not to starve, insisting on the fact that "God is happy with

---

52   ASV, Sant'Uffizio, *Processi: Contro Antonio Massimo medico*, B. 32; see the deposition a woman called Lucia gave on October 29, 1560.

53   "Se ne è andato in Oderzo vostro casal e gli se ne è acasato che fosse la città più tenero terreno," ASV, Sant'Uffizio, *Processi: Contro Antonio Massimo medico*, B. 32, undated.

54   Jean-Pierre Gaberel, *Histoire de l'église de Genève*, vol. 1 (Geneva, 1855), 174.

55   On the role and the characteristics of early modern Italian *medici condotti*, see Richard Palmer, "Physicians and the State in Post-Medieval Italy," in Andrew Russell, ed., *The Town and State Physician from the Middle Ages to Enlightenment* (Wolfenbüttel, 1981), 47-61.

people's work, as much as with them going to mass."[56] Moreover, he proved his evangelical and charitable conception of Christianity by buying meat to feed all the sick in Gardone. Arrested in 1550, De Giusti soon accepted to recant.[57] Due to his willingness to collaborate his sentence was light. Nonetheless, the judges imposed that he retracted both in Venice and in Gardone in front of his fellow villagers and would-be patients.

The case of De Giusti was not exceptional. Mixing popular and erudite elements, socio-economic and spiritual claims, Anabaptism attracted many physicians – like Niccolò Buccella or Lorenzo Tizzano, alias Benedetto Florio, a medical student in Padua.[58] As Aldo Stella has shown, Venetian Anabaptism absorbed the radical views that inspired the German Peasants' War, thanks to the mediation of the Tyrolese refugees who crossed the border after that the rebellion was repressed.[59] Moreover, as a result of the "Anabaptists council" that took place in Venice in 1550, the movement embraced the very radical doctrines put forward by the Neapolitan Valdesians who migrated to the Republic.[60] The charitable attitude typical of the radical branches of the Reformation possibly matched the ethical sensitivity of many Italian medical doctors, whereas the daring doctrinal speculations put forward by the Valdesians (on whether Jesus Christ was divine or human in nature, or whether one had to believe Mary's virginity) appealed to men of culture accustomed to a philological, rational interpretation of the Scriptures.[61] Generally speaking, in fact, most heretical physicians held positions that did not fit into any of the existing denominations of Christianity, which was *per se* dangerous from the point of view of the Inquisition.

---

56   "Istendo in necessità la faria meglio lavorar che andar a messa perche Dio ha aggrato anco del suo lavor quanto del andar a messa," ASV, Sant'Uffizio, *Processi: Contro Stephano medico de Gardon*, B. 8; De Giusti's interrogatory dated November 17, 1550.

57   ASV, Sant'Uffizio, *Processi: Contro Stephano medico de Gardon*, B. 8, dated December 13, 1550.

58   Aldo Stella, *Dall'anabattismo al socinianesimo nel Cinquecento veneto: Ricerche storiche* (Padua, 1967), 121-143; Caccamo, *Eretici italiani*, 51-60; idem in *Dizionario biografico degli Italiani*, vol. 14 (1972), s.v. "Buccella, Niccolò", 750-752; Joanna Kostylo, *Medicine and Dissent in Reformation Europe* (Oxford, forthcoming). Mario Biagioni and Lucia Felici, *La riforma radicale nell'Europa del Cinquecento* (Rome and Bari, 2012), 80.

59   Stella, *Dall'anabattismo al socinianesimo*, 14ff.

60   On the radical Valdesians see Luca Addante, *Eretici e libertini nel Cinquecento italiano* (Rome and Bari, 2010), on the Venetian Anabaptist council, 108-110.

61   On the significance of the concept of *caritas* in Christian medicine, see Jole Agrimi and Chiara Crisciani, "Carità e assistenza."

Therapeutics also enabled learned doctors, as much as other healing figures, to spread heresy in potentially highly receptive environments like hospitals. These had been founded as sacred places for the poor and the sick, and were conceived as spaces in which the patient could enjoy a healthy environment, both from spiritual and physical points of view.[62] Arguably, then, the reception of heterodox ideas inside a hospital environment was due precisely to the highly religious atmosphere which pervaded these places, to the conditions of suffering, anguish and isolation in which the inpatients lived. The persistence of heretical ideas inside the Venetian Hospital for the Incurable and the Hospital of the *Derelitti* in the second half of the sixteenth century suggests that these institutions, a product of Catholic action and devotion, could paradoxically become suitable spaces for the spread of heretical doctrines.[63] Here, the theme of salvation was omnipresent, fuelling a special attention to the spiritual dimension, often in a way that radically diverged from the Counter-Reformation discourse.

The *barbier agli incurabili* Zanetto Cipolla passed religious non-conformist doctrines on to desperately poor and 'incurable' patients at the hospital, gathering them in front of the hearth at night. Being an unlearned surgeon (who had been raised in the hospital as an orphan), Cipolla belonged to a different social class compared to most of the characters I am analysing here. It was probably for this reason that he used to divulge his ideas by focussing on socio-economical claims as much as on doctrinal issues. For instance, he used to argue that priests should give food to the patients at the hospital rather than wake them up in the early morning in order to gather them for mass; or that priests were deceiving the poor regarding the evangelical doctrine in order to steal money from them.[64] His heterodox propaganda, his continuous outpourings of hostility towards the Catholic rituals performed in the hospital, and his refusal to admit his crimes prompted a one-year long trial, which resulted in a severe sentence. Cipolla had to publicly recant at the hospital, apologising to the inpatients that he had scandalised; in addition, he was to attend mass twice a week for five years, and pray the rosary in front of an image of the Virgin Mary every Saturday.

---

62   John Henderson, Horden Peregrine and Alessandro Pastore, eds., *The Impact of Hospitals, 300-2000* (Bern, 2007), 34.

63   On Venetian hospitals, see Bernard Aikema and Dulcia Meijers, eds., *Nel regno dei poveri: Arte e storia dei grandi ospedali veneziani in età moderna, 1474-1797* (Venice, 1989), particularly Richard Palmer, "L'assistenza medica nella Venezia cinquecentesca," 35-42.

64   ASV, *Sant'Uffizio, Processi: Contro Zanetto Barberotto*, B. 23, depositions given on February 4 and on March 10, 1568, respectively by Giorgio Veneto and Augustin di Zuan Battista; the former was in the hospital because he was sick, the latter because he was poor.

The case of the *speziale* Francesco Castellano, who ran the apothecary at the *Derelitti* hospital in Venice, went in a similar direction.[65] What is most interesting about his case is the *speziale*'s radicalism, which led him to assert that there only existed "one law" of God, which worked for Jews, Muslims, Protestants and Catholics.[66] In asserting that there only existed one God, praying to whom was sufficient in order to be safe, Castellano shared the same conception embraced by other heretics from a medical context, who came from different cultural backgrounds, ranging from the *barbiere* Zanetto Cipolla, to the afore mentioned learned doctor Girolamo Donzellini, and to the alchemist Claudio Textor[67] and many others, who, led by their rationalistic approach to the sacred, ended up overcoming all religious denominations. As I have already pointed out, medical radicalism did not match the disciplining ambition of the Roman Church. This contributed to creating a rift between the medical *milieux* and the ecclesiastical authorities, possibly fuelling the reputation of physicians as incorrigible atheists.

---

65 ASV, *Sant'Uffizio, Processi: Contro Francesco Castellano*, B. 32. As archive sources show, in the sixteenth century apothecaries and barbers' shops were important centres for scientific and the religious debates and contributed to the spread of heterodox ideas. See Federico Barbierato, "Dissenso religioso, discussione politica e mercato dell'informazione a Venezia fra seicento e settecento," *Società e storia*, 102 (2003), 707-757; Filippo De Vivo, "Pharmacies as Centres of Communication in Early Modern Venice," in Sandra Cavallo and David Gentilcore, eds., *Spaces, Objects and Identities in Early Modern Italian Medicine* (Hoboken, NJ, 2007), 505-521.

66 "Non intendeva tante leggi, di cristiani ebrei turchi ecc, Dio doveva fare una sola legge," ASV, Sant'Uffizio, *Processi: Contro Francesco Castellano*, B. 32.

67 "L'ho udito anche a dir che non bisognava adorar tanti santi ma che bastava adorar un solo Dio," ASV, Sant'Uffizio, *Processi: Contro Zanetto Barberotto*, B. 23, deposition of Augustin di Zuan Battista, March 12, 1569. In his treatise on anger (published in 1586, one year before the author was executed by the Inquisition), Donzellini maintained that: "Arbitramur enim unam solam, ac veram philosophiam esse, cum vera ac germana religione penitus consentientem, cuius finis sit veritas sincera Dei congnitio & cultus." Girolamo Donzellini, *Remedium ferendarum iniuriarum sive de compescenda ira* (Venice, 1586), f. 2r. For information about the French alchemist Claudio Textor, who was put on trial twice by the Inquisition and sentenced to death in 1587, see ASV, Sant'Uffizio, *Processi: Contro Claudio Textor Francese*, B. 59. According to Aldo Stella, *Dall'anabattismo al socinianesimo*, 159-185, although close to Calvinist doctrines, Textor was not a partisan of any religious denomination, claiming that: "A me basta che si creda in un solo Dio."

Conclusions

By analysing the range of charges brought against Venetian physicians, and examining the texts of their recantations, we can reconstruct how, why and to what extent medical doctors committed religious crimes and attracted the attention of ecclesiastical authorities. There were specific spheres of people's lives and opinions that Inquisition judges thought it was their duty to inquire into; physicians' activities fell into all of them. The possession and distribution of prohibited books was the most common charge among physicians, which is unsurprising since medical doctors were men of culture. The expression of non-conformist religious ideas and/or the doubting of canonical interpretation, aimed at revealing the original meaning of the Holy Scripture, were widespread charges, too. This may, again, be explained with the physicians' intellectual *habitus*. Finally, conscious and often radical propaganda activity was certainly what scared the ecclesiastical authorities the most, and what represented the most serious charge to be faced by the accused during trials. Because of their intellectual and social roles in the community, doctors were, indeed, very well-positioned to spread non-conformist religious views. In some cases, physicians were also put on trial for faults directly related to their professional practice, like ignoring the Church's instructions expressed in the *Super gregem dominicum* papal bull, which was perceived as being opposed to the medical mission.

There was an intellectual proximity between medicine and heresy: the philological accuracy applied by physicians to the texts of Hippocrates and Galen could go hand in hand with the emphasis that the Reformation put on the concept of *sola scriptura* and on the biblical exegesis practice. Furthermore, healing the body and healing the soul continued to be understood as identical missions throughout the century. This conception, already typical of medieval Christian medicine, was emphasised in the sixteenth century by the re-discovery of the Galenic conception of philosophy as the medicine of the soul. This implied that the philosopher-physicians were supposed to deal with both the sacred and the profane. Physicians were often inclined to transferring humanistic lessons from medicine to theology, especially in contexts (such as the Venetian one) where the religious Reformation took root easily. In times of religious crisis, physicians found themselves involved in the theological debate and contributed to making it more radical, as they were used to theological and philosophical speculation. And they stayed firm in their tendency to elude the control of the Church, as long as their professional practice and deontology were concerned. This proved to be a long-lasting feature of medical *milieux* in early modern and modern Venice, in Italy in general, and beyond.

Medicine and the Inquisition in Portugal (Sixteenth and Seventeenth Centuries): People and Books

Hervé Baudry
CHAM, FCSH, Universidade Nova de Lisboa
hbaudry@fcsh.unl.pt

Abstract

The Tribunal of the Inquisition was established in Portugal in 1536. This paper deals with three aspects concerning medicine in sixteenth- and seventeenth-century Portugal: the institution and its members, the medical practitioners, and the books. On the one hand, doctors were necessary to carry out specific duties in the life of the Inquisition. On the other hand, a significant percentage of the victims of the Inquisition were medical professionals, the overwhelming majority being New Christians accused of Judaism. Finally, as did the Roman and Spanish Inquisitions, the Portuguese Holy Office looked after the censorship of books, many of which dealt with medical matters.

Keywords

Portuguese Inquisition – censorship – medicine – Jewish physicians – new Christians – magic

•••

> Monitoring and safeguarding
> are an excellent medicine.
>
> CRASTO[1]

∴

---

* CHAM, Centro de Humanidades, NOVA FCSH – UAC, Av. de Berna 26, 1069-061, Lisboa, Portugal.

1 "Vigiar e acautelar/é mui boa medicina" (António Serrão de Crasto, *Os Ratos da Inquisição* (Porto, 1883), 199). I would like to thank Dr Peter Bull (Sheffield University) and Anke Timmermann for their valued help in improving this article.

The Inquisition was established in Portugal on 23 May 1536 by Pope Paul III through the bull *Cum nihil ad magis*, fifty-eight years after the foundation of the Spanish Inquisition and six years before the Inquisition was re-founded in Rome. Its activities began with the first trials the same year. Tribunals were located in various cities, provoking some reactions of opposition. The Inquisition was not fully functioning until 1565, when three regional tribunals were established, in Coimbra, Évora (a large part of the buildings at Coimbra and Évora still exists) and Lisbon.[2] The capital also had inquisitorial jurisdiction over the territories of the Empire (Africa and Brazil), except Goa (India), where a tribunal was installed in 1560. Some elements specifically contextualize the Portuguese Inquisition in relation to the Spanish one, of whose experience it could take advantage, like the stronger political centralization of the Kingdom and a major participation of the civil authorities in matters of censorship. But it remained autonomous during the period of the Dual Monarchy, that is, the Spanish domination of Portugal (1580-1640). The Portuguese Inquisition was finally abolished in 1821.[3]

The Inquisition was, of course, essentially concerned with theological and religious matters. According to the *Monitório* of November 1536 by the first Inquisitor General Dom Diogo da Silva, Bishop of Ceuta, the crimes to be prosecuted were Judaism, Lutheranism, Islamism, heretical propositions and witchcraft. In the first case, which was by far the most frequent, the victims were New Christians (i.e., forcibly converted Jews and their descendants). No fewer than 45,317 trials are recorded.[4] Building on such archival evidence and on a rapidly growing body of scholarship, the aim of this article is to provide an overview of the complex, manifold relationship between the Inquisition, pervasive as it was, and medicine in early modern Portugal, in terms of both compliance and repression. Although, as we shall see, the Inquisition was mainly interested in tackling Jewish practitioners, it nonetheless needed medical staff to carry out various tasks. Furthermore, it was in charge of the censorship of books. Today Portuguese libraries still own a large number of copies bearing evidence of this censorship.

---

2   On the early decades of the Portuguese Inquisition, see Giuseppe Marcocci and José Paiva, *História da Inquisição Portuguesa* (Lisbon, 2013), 33-43.

3   Francisco Bethencourt, *História das Inquisições: Portugal, Espanha, Itália* (Lisbon, 1996), 22-39; Marcocci and Paiva, *História*, 29-45; Ana Isabel López-Salazar Codes, "O Santo Ofício no tempo dos Filipes: Transformações institucionais e relações de poder," *Revista de história da sociedade e da cultura*, 9 (2009), 147-161. The Inquisition of Goa was abolished in 1812.

4   Of which 13,667 by the Inquisition of Goa (Marcocci and Paiva, *História*, 12).

Some Preliminary Remarks on the Medical Vision of the Inquisition

It should first be remembered that the Inquisition was often compared to medicine, and the inquisitors to physicians. According to the bull of 1536, the Portuguese Inquisition was instituted against heresy, "so that such plagues do not extend their harmful poisons to others."[5]

The Portuguese Inquisition was the local response of the Catholic Church to what was perceived a universal danger that increased with the introduction of the printed book, a dangerous agent of contagion. This vision of heresy as a mortal and contagious disease goes back to the early Church. Jerome, a Father of the Church, and Thomas Aquinas are commonly quoted in this respect as well as Gratian's *Decretum* and the *Decretales*. The heretic is a sick person who needs to be cured, and the inquisitors are the physicians able to achieve this task. Censorship decontaminates the texts through operations referred to with the metaphorical verbs *resecare* or *purgare*. The theologian Nicolaus Eymerich provided a major work of reference for the Iberian inquisitors: his *Directorium Inquisitorum* (written ca. 1376) had first been printed in 1503 in Barcelona. A later commentator, Francisco Peña, added passages on this medical concept. In the preface to the second part of the *Directorium*, he writes that acting against heretics requires as firm an attention as does healing or navigating; a physician not only conserves health, but also explains the nature and types of diseases in order to expel them.[6] The preface to part three is entirely dedicated to this concept. Beginning with a reflection on the marvellous perfection of the human body, Peña compares heresy to a serious humoral disorder, a wound without remedy (*"immedicabile vulnus"*) that needs to be cut into the flesh, and heretics to incurable plague patients (*"pestilentes incurabiles"*), referring to Ovid. Eymerich, a "physician of the Christian Republic," instructs the judge inquisitors who are doctors trained to cure and eradicate the heresy.[7] For Luís de

---

5   Visconde de Santarém, *Corpo diplomatico portuguez*, vol. 3 (Lisbon, 1868), 303: "ne huiusmodi pestes in pernitiem aliorum sua venena difundant."

6   Nicolau Eymerich and Francisco Peña, *Directorium Inquisitorum* (Rome, 1585), 56: "Hoc enim spectat in qualibet arte ad peritum prudentem artificem […][.] Neque medicus solam sanitatem tuetur […], sed idem morbos generaque morborum et naturam explicat, ut vitentur et fugiantur."

7   Ibid., 416: "sunt ad curandam et avellendam haeresim medici." The reference is to Ovid, *Metamorphoses*, I, 190-191.

Páramo, who wrote a successful book on the Holy Office, punishment is a medicine.[8]

In a nutshell, in the Christian vision, heresy is a spiritual disease (*"morbus animi"*) which can be cured by physical means. The first *Regimento da Santa Inquisiçao* (1552) states that the inquisitors should attempt to grant the soul a remedy by salvation rather than punish with the full force of the law.[9] According to António de Sousa, the author of the *Aphorismi Inquisitorum*, punishment should be a medicine more than a poison.[10] Likewise, the famous *Tratado sobre os varios meyos, que se offerecerão a sua Magestade Catholica para remedio do judaismo neste Reyno de Portugal*, by the Inquisitor General Fernão Martins Mascarenhas, discusses the means by which to remedy the Jewish infection in Portugal, and must be understood in this same medico-political perspective.[11]

The medical metaphor was so common that, in the early decades of the Portuguese Inquisition, Samuel Usque referred to such a therapeutic vision ironically: "although one hardly cures one disease with another, this kind of medicine was approved by those excellent lords whose great science supplied us with remedies against the afflictions of the soul."[12] And what is commonly said for individuals is also valid for books: heretical writings are poison, and the authorities must apply for antidotes.[13]

The Medical Professionals as Inquisitorial Staff

Whereas inquisitors are, in modern terms, metaphorical professionals of medicine, real medical practitioners were needed in various situations. The Inqui-

---

8   Luís de Páramo, *De origine et progressu Officii Sanctae Inquisitionis, eiusque dignitate et utilitate* (Madrid, 1592), 746: "punitio [...] medicina est."

9   See on this point Paulo de Assunção and José Eduardo Franco, *As metamorfoses de um polvo: Religião e política nos Regimentos da Inquisição portuguesa (séc. XVI-XIX)* (Lisbon, 2004), 110.

10 António de Sousa, *Aphorismi inquisitorum* (Lisbon, 1630), vol. 3, 26, "De poenis arbitrariis communia," f. 277r: "magis medicina quam venenum."

11 Fernão Martins de Mascarenhas, *Tratado sobre os varios meyos, que se offerecerão a sua Magestade Catholica para remedio do judaismo neste Reyno de Portugal* (s.l., [1625?]).

12 Samuel Usque, *Consolacam: As tribulacoens de Ysrael* (Ferrara, 1553), f. 2r: "posto que maamente se cura hum mal com outro todavia este genero de meizinha foi aprovado por aquelles exçelentes barões que com sua muita çiença rremedios pera aflições dalma nos deixaram."

13 Claude Clément, *Musei sive Bibliothecae tam privatae quam publicae extructio, instructio, cura, usus* (Lyon, 1635), 433: "certis pharmacopolis et juratis pigmentariis auctoritate publica licet eiusmodi toxica antidotis componendis idonea asservare."

sition divided its personnel into two categories: ministers (*ministros*) and officials (*oficiais*). In the seventeenth century, physicians, surgeons and barbers were among those in charge of non-theological tasks, like the governors, caretakers and wardens, who were generally laymen. In more general terms, the medical activities of physicians, surgeons, chemists and blood-letters were equated to those of attorneys, lawyers, ship masters and firemen. No mention of their presence can be found in the first *Regimento* of 1552, but the *Regimentos* printed in 1613 and 1640 are increasingly explicit on their status and functions.[14]

The medical staff acting for the Holy Office is listed in 1613 as follows: physicians, surgeons, barbers, midwives and women administrating enemas (*"cristeleiras"*).[15] It is worthy of note that the last two mentioned, whose art was regulated in the city of Lisbon in 1572, would disappear from subsequent *Regimentos*.[16] Apparently none of them were full members of the institution, as they do not appear in the list of the ministers and officials (t. 7-17). In one case, it refers to "the physician of the Holy Office," whose duty was to cure the prisoners (t. 10 c. 18); depending on the prisoner's condition, he should persuade him to confess (t. 4 c. 21). Physicians and surgeons are needed to determine whether a prisoner was murdered or committed suicide (t. 4 c. 31).[17] Everyone enters the building under oath (*"juramento"*) to observe secrecy (t. 6 c. 11) and must be accompanied by the governor of the jail (*"alcade,"* t. 10 c. 19), who had the custody of the keys, if a physician is called out of hours (t. 10 c. 22). Their presence during the sessions of torture is not specified but is well documented before 1613.[18]

The *Regimento* of 1640 remained valid until 1774.[19] The practice of medicine in the inquisitorial facilities had become so institutionalized that a specific volume was published separately, *Regimento do médico, çurgião, e barbeyro*. The main change is that two physicians, one surgeon and one barber, are now salaried as full-time officials. They are at the service of the tribunal to cure the prisoners, the members of the Inquisition and their parents (l. 1, t. 1; t. 20 §4),

---

14   *Regimento*, 1552, in Assunção and Franco, *As metamorfoses*, 109-135.

15   *Regimento*, 1613, ibid., 151-227.

16   Vergílio Correia, *Livro dos Regimentos dos oficiaes mecanicos da mui nobre e sempre leal cidade de Lisboa (1572)* (Coimbra, 1926), chs. 71, 72.

17   Cases of suicide are discussed in Isabel Drumond Braga, *Viver e morrer nos cárceres da Inquisição* (Lisbon, 2015), 175-176.

18   Elvira Cunha de Azevedo Mea, *A Inquisição de Coimbra no século XVI: A instituição, os homens e a sociedade* (Porto, 1997), 153, 469-474, 696.

19   On these general dispositions, see Ana C. de Faria, *O Regimento de 1640 e a justiça inquisitorial portuguesa: "Conforme a melhor e mais segura opinião e estilo do Sancto Officio"* (Coimbra, 2016).

and are recruited from the local elite (§1, *"os mais sufficientes que ouver na terra"*).[20] For instance, in Goa, a *"pandite,"* an Indian physician, was called to cure Charles Dellon, a French physician who had been arrested, and feigned sickness with the aim of committing suicide by means of excessive blood-letting.[21] Some differences appear in the question of the confession: the physician now only informs the inquisitor about the necessity to provide a dying prisoner with the opportunity to confess (l. 1 t. 14 §14), whereas the previous *Regimento* gave him more discretion.[22] He is not to be informed of the degree of torture to which an accused was submitted (l. 2 t. 13 §5) but was to decide whether the accused could be submitted to torture depending on his health condition (l. 2 t. 13 §5).[23] Any death had to be certified, and in each case a death certificate (*auto da morte*) established, i.e. whether it had been a natural or a violent death (l. 2 t. 17 §2; t. 18 §1). Although this was not specified, we may also assume that the physicians' expertise was called upon in cases of madness, both actual or feigned (l. 2 t. 17 §1).[24]

As Federico Barbierato stated in the Venetian case, "the use of forensic medicine by the tribunal was mostly a routine."[25] However, in some cases it was critical, as is shown by the following examples: João Freixo, an Old Christian imprisoned as a Jew, was released after proving that he had been circumcised for medical reasons. João Bravo Chamisso testified that the physical state of António Homem did not preclude his capacity to sodomize. Due to a certified dropsy, Pedro Duarte Ferrão escaped the *auto de fé* ('Act of Faith,' which refers to the ritual of public penance of condemned heretics and apostates) in Lisbon in May 1682.[26]

---

20   *Regimento do médico, çurgião, e barbeyro*, [s.d], Biblioteca Nacional de Portugal, Cod. 867; *Regimento*, 1640 (in Assunção and Franco, *As metamorfoses*, 233-418); Braga, *Viver*, 143-176.

21   Charles Dellon, *Relation de l'Inquisition de Goa* (Paris, 1688), 214-217.

22   Of course, the Council of Trent had reinstated that the moral ultimate requirement of the medical profession was to save the soul of the sick, see O. di Simplicio, "Medicina," in Adriano Prosperi, ed., *Dizionario storico dell'Inquisizione*, vol. 2 (Pisa, 2010), 1014-1015.

23   There were seven or ten degrees of torture, from facing the instrument (*polé* or *potro*) to the most painful action, see Isaías da Rosa Pereira, *Documentos para a história da Inquisição* (Porto, 1984), 109-112; Mea, *A Inquisição*, 469-471.

24   Mea, *A Inquisição*, 424; on the activities of the Inquisition's *médico dos cárceres*, see Timothy D. Walker, *Doctors, Folk Medicine and the Inquisition: The Repression of Magical Healing in Portugal During the Enlightenment* (The Hague, 2005), 180-208.

25   Federico Barbierato, "Les corps comme preuve: Médecins et inquisiteurs dans les pratiques judiciaires du Saint-Office," *L'Atelier du Centre de recherches historiques* (<http://acrh.revues.org/5223; DOI: 10.4000/acrh.5223>, accessed April 21, 2018).

26   See, respectively, Arquivo Nacional da Torre do Tombo, Inquisição de Lisboa, processo n.º 18023 (henceforth, ANTT, Inq. Évora or Lisboa or Coimbra, proc.); ANTT, Inq. Lisboa, proc. 15421, 264; ANTT, Inq. Lisboa, proc. 8096, f. 217r.

An auxiliary category was that of the familiars of the Holy Office. They were members of civil society who assisted the actions of the tribunals, such as arresting the suspects, leading them to prison, or confiscating their assets. It added prestige and resulted in privileges.[27] It was no coincidence that João Curvo Semedo, a physician from Monforte, highlighted his status on the title page of his medical works.[28] Not everyone could join the Holy Office, a point which refers to its fundamental scope: the fight against Judaism. Providing evidence for the purity of one's blood (*limpeza de sangue*) was compulsory. A legal diploma (*habilitação*) was delivered after an inquiry which proved that the candidate's parents were not of Jewish origin. The same Old Christian genealogy was required from the fellows of medicine (*porcionistas*) at the University of Coimbra, who were under the protection of the King: they "cannot be of Jewish, New Christian, or Moorish origin, nor even of infamous origin or have a communicable disease."[29]

The Medical Professionals, Victims of the Inquisition Like Others

The activity of the Inquisition in matters of medicine is closely linked to the repression of Judaism in Portugal following the royal decree issued in December 1496. We have no statistics about the distribution of medical professionals between Old and New Christians, for example among the students of medicine at the University of Coimbra who represented 6.9% of the total of students registered during the period 1573-1772.[30] Medical professionals represent about

---

27   On the familiars in Spain and Portugal, see Bethencourt, *História*, 47-50; Bruno Lopes, "Familiares do Santo Ofício, população e estatuto social (Évora, primeira metade de setecentos)," in *I congresso histórico internacional: As cidades na história: População*, vol. 3, 2 (Guimarães, 2013), 279-308, and Walker's chapter in this volume.

28   João Curvo Semedo, *Tratado da peste* (Lisbon, 1680), and *Polyanthea medicinal* (Lisbon, 1697): both title pages qualify the author as "medico, familiar do Santo Officio, e cavalleyro professo da Ordem de Christo." Likewise, Francisco Morato Roma highlights his position of "medico do Santo Officio" in his *Luz da medicina* (Lisbon, 1664).

29   *Regimento dos medicos e barbeiros christãos velhos* (s.l., 1604), 1: "Os que ouverem de ser admitidos ao partido da Medicina, não hão de ser raça de Judeu, Christão novo, nem Mouro, nem proceder de gente infame, nem ter doenças contagiosas." These measures were first taken by King D. Sebastião in 1568, see Francis A. Dutra, "The Practice of Medicine in Early Modern Portugal: The Role and Social Status of the *Físico-mor* and the *Surgião-mor*," in Israel J. Katz *et al.*, eds., *Libraries, History, Diplomacy, and the Performing Arts: Essays in Honor of Carleton Sprague Smith* (New York, NY, 1991), 135-169, 139-140.

30   António Borges Coelho, "Tópicos para o estudo da relação Universidade-Inquisição (mea-

5% of the total of those accused by the Inquisition of Évora,[31] 3% in the initial decades of the Inquisition of Lisbon.[32] The great majority of them were New Christians, that is, Jews converted by force to Christianity in 1497, when the community might total between 3%[33] and 10%[34] of the estimated population of one million inhabitants of Portugal.[35] Besides all estimations, the physicians, at least in the fifteenth century, were Jewish in majority.[36]

The *Aphorismi Inquisitorum* report prohibitions regarding Christians: they may not consult Jewish physicians except in case of extreme necessity and must not buy from or sell remedies to them.[37] As for New Christians, although they were not admitted as *porcionistas*, they did have the possibility to be admitted to the University.[38] For instance, Pedro Rebelo, a New Christian later accused of Judaism, was trained there in medicine.[39] Ten out of the eleven trials against students involve New Christians.[40] Various famous teachers were New Christians, at least in the sixteenth century, such as António Luís (d. 1565,

dos XVI-meados XVII)," *Universidade(s): História, memória, perspectivas*, 4 (Coimbra, 1991), 257-270, 264.

31   To be exact, 4.9% according to Michèle Janin-Tivos Tailland, *Inquisition et société au Portugal: La cas du tribunal d'Évora, 1660-1821* (Paris, 2001), 187; and 5.9% according António Borges Coelho, *Inquisição de Évora* (Lisbon, 1987), vol. 1, 382. In Lisbon during the initial four decades, the percentage amounted to 3%: Daniel Norte Giebels, *A Inquisição de Lisboa: No epicentro da dinâmica inquisitorial (1537-1579)* (Coimbra, 2016), 241.

32   Giebels, *A Inquisição*, 241.

33   Maria José P.F. Tavares, *Os Judeus em Portugal no século XV* (Lisbon, 1982), 74.

34   Israel S. Révah, "Entrevista com o Prof. I.S. Révah conduzida por Abílio Diniz Silva," *Diario de Lisboa*, 6 May 1971, 2-4; António J. Saraiva, *Inquisição e Cristãos-novos* (Lisbon, 1994), 216.

35   João J. Alves Dias, "A População," in Joel Serrão and A.H. de Oliveira Marques, eds., *Nova história de Portugal*, vol. 5 (Lisbon, 1998), 11-15. On the presence of Jews from Spain after the establishment of the Inquisition, see François Soyer, *The Persecution of the Jews and Muslims of Portugal* (Leiden, 2007), 104-105.

36   Iria Gonçalves, "Físicos e cirurgiões quatrocentistas: As cartas de exame," *Do tempo e da história*, vol. 1 (Lisbon, 1965), 69-112, 84. On the Jews and medicine, see Lúcia L. Mucznik et al., eds., *Dicionário do judaísmo português* (Barcarena, 2009), 349-355.

37   Sousa, *Aphorismi*, I, 36, §§8-9.

38   The University, including the Faculty of Medicine, left Lisbon for Coimbra one year after the establishment of the Inquisition. On the "common Jewish background" of its professors, see Mário Farelo, "Garcia de Orta, the Faculty of Medicine at Lisbon, and the Portuguese Overseas Endeavor at the Beginning of the Sixteenth Century," *Journal of Medieval Iberian Studies*, 7 (2015), 218-231.

39   ANTT, Inq. Lisboa, proc. 2676.

40   ANTT, Inq. Coimbra, proc. 967, 1344, 3262, 3469, 6676, 10188; ANTT, Inq. Lisboa, proc. 3389, 7781,10267; ANTT, Inq. Évora, proc. 11426.

who was imprisoned for one week in Lisbon in 1539), Tomás Rodrigues da Veiga (1513-1579), Ambrósio Nunes (1529-1611), or Francisco Carlos (M.D. in 1560)[41].

Arguably, the repression of New Christian medics was inspired by personal interests from "old enemies with scores to settle," as was the case for the physician of Lamego, Pedro Furtado, in the early 1540s; considering that trials were launched after denunciations, professional competition must have played a part.[42] Manuel Soares Brandão, who was arrested in 1702, complained that he was a victim of his colleagues' revenge.[43] According to Warren Anderson, who has quantified the condemnations in Évora and Lisbon between 1635 and 1763, "poor folk healers and New Christian medics were arrested for competing with Old Christian doctors. As Old Christians gained more power, they eliminated more of their competition with the support of the crown and Inquisitor General."[44] Walker has shown the collaboration between the doctors of Coimbra and the Inquisition in the case of the popular healers.[45]

Statistics prove the near exclusivity of the anti-Judaic policies in the Portuguese Inquisition. The table shown here gives an overview of the trials both for male practitioners (physicians, surgeons, barbers, students of medicine and chemists) and female practitioners (midwives and women administrating enemas).[46] One category is set apart, that of folk healers, for which trials are infrequent in our period.[47]

The Portuguese Inquisition harshly repressed the practice of Judaism, whether suspected or proved, among the New Christians; incidentally, only one of the accused in our list, Isaac Almosnino, is identified as being a Jew.[48] Coelho, through the analysis of 8,210 processes, established that the 'hunting

---

41   On Veiga, see Lígia Bellini, "Notes on Medical Scholarship and the Broad Intellectual Milieu in Sixteenth-Century Portugal," *Portuguese Studies*, 15 (1999), 11-41, 16.

42   Susana B. Mateus and James W. Nelson Novoa, "The Case of the New Christians of Lamego as an Example of Resistance against the Portuguese Inquisition in Sixteenth-Century Portugal," *Hispana Judaica*, 6 (2008), 83-103, 88-95; José P. Paiva, *Bruxaria e superstição num país sem "caça às bruxas": 1600-1774* (Lisbon, 2002), 208.

43   ANTT, Inq. Lisboa, proc. 2110, f. 9r.

44   R. Warren Anderson, "Inquisitorial Punishments in Lisbon and Évora," *Journal of Portuguese History*, 10 (2012), 19-36, 52.

45   Walker, *Doctors*, 202-208.

46   The table is based on search results from the online catalog of the Portuguese National Archives, using the following search criteria: period <1536-1700>, terms of professional categories: físico, médico, cirurgião, barbeiro, sangrador, boticário, parteira, criste.a.leira, curandeiro/a.

47   On this point, see Walker, *Doctors*, 25-31.

48   ANTT, Inq. Lisboa, proc. 5393, 12799.

TABLE 1   *Percentage of medical professionals condemned for Judaism (1536-1700)*

Professional category	Number of trials	Condemned for Judaism[a]	Percentage of Condemnations
médicos, físicos	159[b]	133	83,6
cirurgiões	100[c]	66	66
sangradores	5	5	71,4
boticários	89	79	88,8
parteiras, cristaleiras[d]	10	5	50
TOTAL	365[e]	288	78,9
Other categories			
curandeiro	17	0	0
curandeira	10	0	0

a   Prosecution on account of Judaism and apostasy or heresy, the last applying when the accused was a New Christian.
b   Of which 11 were students.
c   Of which 2 were apprentices.
d   On births in jails, see Braga, *Viver*, ch. 6. We did not encounter either female nurses (*"enfermeira de mulheres"* in the *Regimento* of the hospital Todos-os-Santos, Lisbon) or male ones in the criminal records. In two cases, the fathers of both of the accused were nurses (ANTT, Inq. Lisboa, proc. 13144; ANTT, Inq. Évora, proc. 8691). On Moorish and Jewish women healers in Spain, see Leigh Whaley, *Women and the Practice of Medical Care in Early Modern Europe, 1400-1800* (London, 2011), 147-149.
e   Number of processes per tribunal: Lisbon, 177 (48.5%); Évora, 126 (34.5%); Coimbra, 61 (17%).

ground' of the Inquisition of Évora during a century and a half dealt with Judaism and apostasy in 89% of cases.[49] In Lisbon and Coimbra this number was, respectively, 68% and 83%.[50] As for the other countries, which are not so fully documented, the figures for cases of Judaism and apostasy in Spain range between 1.9% and 18.3%; and, in more fragmentary documentation for Italy (only

---

49   "[T]erreno de caça" (Coelho, *Inquisição*, 185); 81.56% (1660-1821) according to Tailland, *Inquisition*, 247. On the period between 1536 and 1676, see Maria Bendita Araújo, "Médicos e seus familiares na Inquisição de Évora," *Comunicações apresentadas ao 1º congresso Luso-Brasileiro sobre a Inquisição* (Lisbon, 1989), vol. 1, 271-280.
50   Bethencourt, *História*, 279; a lower rate applied to Évora: 84%.

two regions are captured), they are between 2% and 3%.[51] Although incomplete, these numbers highlight the huge difference between Portugal and the other inquisitions, and reflect Portugal's "anti-Judaic obsession."[52] In addition, Anderson delivered clear statistics for the death penalty for the Inquisition of Évora from 1636 to 1778: "Those killed were mostly executed because they were Jewish. The minimum estimate suggests that more than 80% were alleged crypto-Jews and the maximum estimate points to more than 95%."[53] Even the dead could be physically eliminated, like the reputed physician and naturalist Garcia de Orta (d. 1568, Goa), whose corpse was exhumed and burned in 1580.[54]

As regards other crimes of which medical professionals were accused, in the early stages of the Inquisition, the physicians to the King seem to have been a particular target for the inquisitors, who were clearly seeking to establish their authority: António de Viseu was imprisoned in 1538 for heresy;[55] in 1539, in a more famous case, the *físico-mor* Aires Vaz did not escape prosecution for witchcraft (*bruxaria*, corresponding in his case to judicial astrology);[56] and Dionísio was burnt *in effigie* in 1541.[57]

---

51   Ibid., 270-271. In Naples, the range was 2% to 6%.

52   "Obsessão antijudaica e repressão dos cristãos-novos » (Marcocci and Paiva, *História*, title of ch. 2, p. 49, my translation). For the Spanish and Portuguese physicians' social approach, see Jon Arrizabalaga, "The World of Iberian *converso* Practitioners, from Lluís Alcanyís to Isaac Cardoso," in Víctor Navarro and William Eamon, eds., *Más allá de la leyenda negra: España y la revolución científica / Beyond the Black Legend: Spain and the Scientific Revolution* (Valencia, 2007), 307-322.

53   Anderson, "Inquisitorial Punishments," 29.

54   *Regimento*, 1613, t. 4 c. 27; 1640, l. 2 t. 26. Jon Arrizabalaga, "Garcia de Orta in the Context of the Sephardic Diaspora," in Palmira Fontes da Costa, ed., *Medicine, Trade and Empire: Garcia de Orta's Colloquies on the Simples and Drugs of India (1563) in Context* (Farnham, 2015), 11-32, 18-20. It should be noted that Orta's printer, João de Endem, was the printer for the first Archbishop of Goa, D. Gaspar Leão Pereira. The latter had arrived in India in 1560, followed by the responsibles for the establishment of the Inquisition and two printing presses (Maria Teresa Carvalho, *O mundo natural asiático aos olhos do Ocidente*, PhD dissertation, Lisbon University, 2012, 106-107). In 1565 Endem also printed the *Tratado que fez mestre Hieronimo Medico do papa Benedicto 13 contra os Judeus*, a translation into Portuguese of the anti-Judaic treatise by Jerónimo de Santa Fé (1411), a *converso* physician for the Antipope Benedict XIII.

55   ANTT, Inq. Lisboa, proc. 7816.

56   ANTT, Inq. Lisboa, proc. 13186. See Alexandre Herculano, *História da origem e estabelecimento da Inquisição* (Lisbon, 1975), t. 2, 195-196 (Herculano gives evidence that Vaz was a New Christian); Marcocci and Paiva, *História*, 34-35.

57   António L. Andrade, "Ciência, religião e livros na Europa de quinhentos: A controvérsia da sangria entre Pierre Brissot e Dionísio Brudo," *Cadernos de estudos sefarditas*, 14 (2015), 127-129.

More generally, Table 2 provides a tentative survey of the processes, in the decreasing order of the number of processes counted in brackets ("NC" means New Christian).

TABLE 2   *Medical delinquency according to the Portuguese Inquisition (1536-1700)*

Crime	Surgeons	Physicians
bigamia	4 (3 NC)	1 (NC)
poligamia[a]	1	
Luteranismo	4 (2 French, 1 Polish, 1 Portuguese)	1 (NC)
Calvinismo	1 (NC)	1 (German)
Islamismo	1	
Sodomia	3 (2 NC)	2 (NC)
impedir o recto ministério do Sº Ofício (hindrance of the action of the H.O.)	2 (NC)	1 (NC)
quebra do sígilo (violation of secrecy)	1 (NC)	
violação de juramento (violation of oath)	1	
desobediência ao S.O. (disobedience to the H.O.)		1 (NC)
dizer o crime de que for a acusado (reporting the crime you were accused of)		1 (NC)
Sacrilégio	1 (NC)	
Blasfémio	1	3 (1 NC, 1 Jew, 1 Hindu)
heresia (questão das indulgências)	1 (NC)	0
degredo não cumprido (failure to complete deportation)	1 (NC)	0
Perjúrio	1 (NC)	2 (NC)
irreverência	1	1
falsidade	1	0
feitiçaria (illegal healing)	1 (NC)	0
fazer-se passar por cristão-novo (pose as New Christian)	1	0
exercer o seu ofício e andar numa mula de sela (to do one's duty and to ride a saddle mule)	1 (NC)	0
confissão diminuta	0	1 (NC)
enviar escritos ao irmão preso na Inquisição (sending writings to a brother imprisoned by the Inquisition)	0	1
pacto com o diabo (pact with the devil)		1 (Spanish)
bruxaria (witchcraft)		1

a   The accused, Manuel Lopes da Fonseca, married three times (ANTT, Inq. Coimbra, proc. 226).

Some of the medical practitioners who were condemned for Judaism had authored books. Two of them were licenced physicians, Henrique do Quental Vieira (d. 1664) and Simão Pinheiro Morão (1620-1686), the latter imprisoned twice for long periods, in 1656-1659 and in 1667-1675.[58] A professor of mathematics at the University of Coimbra, André de Avelar (1546-*ca.* 1623), joins this group, as his *Repertorio dos tempos*, with editions published between 1585 and 1602, contains a part (book IV) on medical astrology, to which we will return below. He was imprisoned for two weeks in 1620 for Judaism, and again in 1621 for having lapsed, and probably died in prison two years later.[59] Significantly, in none of these cases the inquisitors ever examined the accused's writings.

Mention should be made here of António Serrão de Crasto (or Castro, 1610-*ca.* 1685). A pharmacist in a family of physicians, he was , like Quental Vieira, a member of the *Academia dos singulares* of Lisbon. Arrested in 1672 at the age of 60, he was released, ill and one-eyed, eleven years later.[60] He wrote short poems and, potentially, a 1,880 line poem, *Os Ratos da Inquisição*, during his imprisonment. This text focused on the theme of hunger and was published for the first time by Camilo Castelo Branco, who himself composed his masterpiece, *Amor de perdição*, in jail. Crasto's poem is one of the few known texts of prison literature in early modern Portugal; others are George Buchanan's Latin paraphrase of the Psalms, Cristóvão Falcão's verses in the *Carta do mesmo estando preso*, and the comedies of Gaspar Mendes, a medical student.[61]

Inquisitorial Censorship

The Inquisition not only dealt with human beings, but from 1559 it was also responsible for controlling books. Even more than individuals, inquisitors saw books as powerful agents of contamination of the society.[62] Censorship was a

---

58   ANTT, Inq. Lisboa, proc. 8845. ANTT, Inq. Lisboa, proc. 616 and 616-1. On their works, see "Bibliografia médica lusa (século XVII)," in Hervé Baudry, *Livro médico e censura na primeira modernidade em Portugal* (Lisbon, 2017), Vieira: 101, 114, 136, 156; Morão: 96, 99, 114, 140, 155.

59   ANTT, Inq. Coimbra, proc. 2209 and 2209-1; his four children were also arrested.

60   ANTT, Inq. Lisboa, proc. 4910. He was the second of ten members of his family to be arrested, see Heitor Gomes Teixeira, *As tábuas do painel de um auto (António Serrão de Crasto)* (Lisbon, 1977), 54. One of his sons, Pedro, a medical student in Coimbra and the author of satirical poems, was executed in 1682.

61   Braga, *Viver*, 241-248.

62   On the context of Spanish inquisitorial censorship, see Martin Austin Nesvig, "'Heretical Plagues' and Censorship Cordons: Colonial Mexico and the Transatlantic Book Trade,"

matter of royal and Church control, and in principle shared by the bishops and the inquisitors according to the rules laid down by the *Index librorum prohibitorum* of the Council of Trent (1564). The Portuguese Dominican Francisco Foreiro played an important role in this story.[63] In Portugal the Inquisition, armed with powerful and specific methods, led the operations.[64] The two Iberian Inquisitions, in addition to the Roman rules and lists of prohibited books, produced their own lists, relevant to the local production of writings, and with some legal characteristics.[65]

As in the procedures against people, everyone was subject to social monitoring, from the producer of books (author, printer) to the consumer (reader), and from the bibliographical filtering to denunciations against book owners.[66] In Portugal, the book trade were characterized by a limited local production and extensive imports from Europe, directly to Portugal or via Spain. In this respect, the internal demand for medical books was mostly satisfied by imports. Nonetheless, the local production increased from the sixteenth to the seventeenth century, with the greatest progression happening during the first half of the seventeenth century.[67]

Church History, 75 (2006), 5-8; Enrique Gacto, "Libros venenosos," *Revista de la Inquisición,* 6 (1997), 7-44.

63   See Prosperi, ed., *Dizionario storico,* 613-614.

64   Marcocci and Paiva, *História,* 91-98.

65   "Regras geraes do Catalogo de Portugal acrecentadas às do Catalogo universal Romano" Fernão Martins Mascarenhas, *Index auctorum damnatae memoriae: Tum etiam librorum, qui vel simpliciter, vel ad expurgationem usque prohibentur, vel denique expurgati permittuntur* (Lisbon, 1624), 81-86).

66   Despite the legislation put in place by the Council of Trent, in contrast to the Iberian Inquisitions, the Roman bureaucracy of censorship was not centralized until the end of the sixteenth century. See Gigliola Fragnito, "La censura libraria tra Congregazione dell' Indice, Congregazione dell'Inquisizione e maestro del Sacro Palazzo," in Ugo Rozzo, ed., *La censura libraria nell'Europa del secolo XVI* (Udine, 1997), 163-175.

67   Numbers of items produced in Portugal (by period): 1496-1500: 3; 1501-1550: 7 (+ 133% compared to the previous period); 1551-1600: 12 (+ 71%); 1601-1650: 40 (+ 233%); 1651-1700: 59 (+ 47.5%). On the significance of importations, see Hervé Baudry, "As problemáticas do livro médico em Portugal nos séculos XVI e XVII: Com a bibliografia das obras médicas impressas em Portugal (1496-1598)," in António Andrade, ed., *Do manuscrito ao livro impresso* (Coimbra, forthcoming). On the medical book market in the first half of the seventeenth century, see Hervé Baudry, "Medical Publishing in Portugal in the First Half of the Seventeenth Century: A Good Business?" in Alexander S. Wilkinson and Alejandra Ulla Lorenzo, eds., *A Maturing Market: The Iberian Book World in the First Half of the Seventeenth Century* (Leiden, 2017), p. 225-240.

Two Inquisitors General are worthy of note: Cardinal Dom Henrique (Inquisitor General from 1539 to 1580), and the Bishop of the Algarve Dom Fernão Martins Mascarenhas (from 1616 to 1628). Both left a deep mark on censorship for nearly a century. The first, a brother of the King, quickly implemented measures of control, among which are the earliest Portuguese lists of prohibited books;[68] the second was responsible for the last Portuguese Index of 1624, which remained valid until the abolition of the Holy Office.[69]

Without going into the debate of the efficacy of book control measures in the early modern period, the issue of textual censorship must take into account the legal instrument used to achieve it, i.e. the indexes.[70] Of course, these documents, with their updated lists of names and titles, do not deliver the whole picture of what happened to all texts and books produced at the time, or the way in which medical knowledge was shaped; only trials illuminate the human side of the story. But what is clear is that the strong centralization of the inquisitorial machine, acting in a relatively small and remote territory bordered by another Inquisitorial State, must have permitted a certain efficiency.

Methodologically, censorship can be tackled in two ways: internally, with the contents censored, and externally, through the censorship of objects, a survey of which provides indicators of efficiency. With the exception of the Roman Index, which was universally valid by principle, the local, Spanish and Portuguese indexes show intertextual similarities. For example, the entry for Amato Lusitano in the Portuguese expurgatory of 1624 comes from the Spanish Index of 1612, with some formal differences, whereas the 1612 entry corresponds by 90% to the Roman expurgation Index of 1607, which had been initiated by the censors by 1587 at the latest.[71] Therefore, an evaluation of the extent of the medical items censored in Portugal requires that we proceed in two phases, describing, first, all items listed during our period; and second, items first listed by the Portuguese.

A second feature of the Iberian inquisitorial indexation is that, differently from Rome (where one expurgatory, incomplete, was produced in 1607), the

68   Jesus M. de Bujanda, *Index de l'inquisition Portugaise: 1547, 1551, 1561, 1564, 1581* (Geneva, 1995).

69   *Index auctorum.*

70   For Spain, see Laura Beck Varela, "¿El censor ineficaz? Una lectura histórico-jurídica del índice e libros prohibidos," *Revista jurídica de la Universidad Autonoma de Madrid*, 31 (2015), 71-89.

71   Ugo Baldini and Leen Spruit, eds., *Catholic Church and Modern Science: Documents from the Archives of the Roman Congregations of the Holy Office and the Index*, vol. 1: *The Sixteenth Century* (Vatican City, 2009), 749-768.

censors widely developed a form of micro-censorship, that is, the expurgation of texts. At the end of the sixteenth century specialized Indexes were produced, in seven editions altogether from 1571 (the first expurgatory produced by the University of Leuven) to 1640 (two Portuguese and four Spanish), excluding the counterfeits.[72] Such a censoring process appeared in the Tridentine Index of 1564, which included three classes of items: damned (heretical) authors (class 1); authors, certain works of whom were authorized after expurgation (class 2); and anonymous works (class 3). Some authors, like Erasmus of Rotterdam, flitted between the first and the second classes. Whereas prohibition is a universal measure against all the works by one author, expurgation is a partial prohibition: a text from the second class continued to be prohibited until it was expurgated; the final authorized text is more or less mutilated. Expurgating involved three kinds of textual modifications (later called instructions), by order of frequency: deletion, substitution, and addition. The observation of direct textual censorship imposed on printed (and manuscript) copies and, more widely, the history of the expurgation provide much information on the perception of medicine by the Church authorities.

Medical Authors Listed in the Expurgatories Printed in Portugal

The list of medical works extracted from all expurgatories printed between 1571 and 1640 totals 118 items at most (112 author names, 6 titles). The Portuguese Indexes contribute sixteen names to the list of authors prohibited by ecclesiastical authorities in Europe, the majority of them with medical works to be expurgated:

–   in 1581: Amato Lusitano (*Centuriae, In Dioscoridem*; Joannes Argenterius, *In artem medicinalem Galeni*);

---

72   Benito Arias Montano, *Index expurgatorius librorum qui hoc seculo prodierunt, vel doctrinæ non sanæ erroribus inspersis* (Antwerp, 1571); Inquisição de Portugal, *Catalogo dos livros que se prohibem nestes regnos* (Lisbon, 1581); Gaspar Quiroga, *Index librorum expurgatorum* (Madrid, 1584); Giovanni Maria Guanzelli, *Index librorum expurgandorum in studiosorum gratiam confecti tomus primus* (Rome, 1607); Bernardo de Sandoval y Rojas, *Index librorum prohibitorum et expurgatorum* (Madrid, 1612); *Index auctorum*; Antonio Zapata, *Novus index librorum prohibitorum et expurgatorum* (Sevilla, 1632); Diego Díaz de la Carrera, *Novissimus librorum prohibitorum et expurgandorum index* (Madrid, 1640). On the counterfeits, see Georges Bonnant, "Les index prohibitifs et expurgatoires contrefaits par des protestants au XVIe et au XVIIe siècle," *Bibliothèque d'humanisme et Renaissance*, 31 (1969), 611-640.

–   in 1624: André de Avelar (*Reportorio dos tempos*); Gonçalo Cabreira (*Com-*
    pendio); Thomas Erastus (non-medical works); Andrés Laguna (*Acerca de*
    la materia medicinal); Andreas Libavius (*Alchimia, Commentarii alchimi-*
    ae, Singularium, Tractati physici); Pietro d'Abano (*Conciliator*); Francis-
    cus Rueus (*De gemmis*); Jacobus Rueffus (*De conceptu hominis*); Oliva
    Sabuco (*Nueva filosofia*); Gaspar Cardoso Sequeira (*Thesouro de pru-*
    dentes); Nicolaus Taurellus (*De medica praedictione*); Pedro Hispano
    (*Thesaurus pauperum, Tesouro de pobres*); Johannes Jacobus Wecker
    (*Medicinæ utriusque Syntaxes*, etc.); Theodor Zwinger (*Commentarii in*
    Hippocratem).

The Portuguese censors were not focused exclusively on local authors. Apart
from five Portuguese authors (Amato, Avelar, Cabreira, Hispano, Sequeira:
none of them is deemed heretic), there were four subjects of the Holy Roman
Empire (Erastus, Libavius, Rueus, Taurellus), three Swiss nationals (Rueffus,
Wecker, Zwinger), two Spaniards (Laguna, Sabuco) and two Italians (Argenterius, Pietro d'Abano). Hispano and Pietro d'Abano were actually medieval
authors. Amato Lusitano's widely disseminated *Centuriae* and comment on
Dioscorides were never published in Portugal. The *Thesaurus pauperum*,
whose authorship remained doubtful, was composed during the second half of
the thirteenth century, allegedly by the Portuguese Pedro Hispano (Petrus His-
panus, Pedro Julião, 1215-1277), who was later elected pope under the name of
John XXI.[73] The Index of 1624 expurgated the Latin text and the Spanish translation. Moreover, the same entry includes Gonçalo Cabreira, a surgeon, who
published a collection of remedies derived from this text in Portuguese in 1611,
which appeared in five editions in the seventeenth century and in three in the
eighteenth. In addition to Avelar, whose fate was described earlier, Sequeira
was a mathematician who dedicated a section of his almanac to astrological
medicine. The works of the Spanish authors, Laguna and Sabuco, were also
widely distributed within and outside the Iberian Peninsula. For Sabuco's
work, first edited in Madrid in 1587, there was a printed edition in Portugal with
an expurgated text according to the requirements of the Portuguese censors.[74]
Including Avelar and Sequeira, the total number of medical titles printed in

---

73   *Index auctorum*, 627: "Auctore (si verum est) Petro Hispano, postea Pontifex Joanne 20
     [sic]." See José F. Meirinhos, "O *Tesouro dos pobres* de Pedro Hispano, entre o século XIII e
     a edição de Scribonius em 1576," in António M.L. Andrade *et al.*, eds, *Humanismo, diás-*
     pora e ciência: Séculos XVI e XVII (Porto, 2013), 327-349.

74   Oliva Sabuco, *Nueva filosofia de la naturaleza del hombre* (Braga, 1622); see Baudry, *Biblio-*
     grafia, 122.

Portugal between 1497 and 1700 is 59. Only three of them were submitted to micro-censorship (Avelar, Cabreira, Sequeira).

Whatever the origin of the authors or the works, if they were prohibited subject to expurgation, all were subjected to the same rules, namely both the Tridentine-Roman rules (Index of 1564, rules 2, 5, 7, 8, 9; the *Instructio* in the Index of 1596, *De correctione librorum*, article 2 with its 17 cases provides with the most detailed instructions) and, in our case, also the Portuguese rules (*Index Lusitaniae* of 1624). The rules also applied to any work, whether it was printed or in written in manuscript (*impresso ou de mão*).

A taxonomy of the contents subjected to micro-censorship in the medical books of the Portuguese Indexes can be extracted from the total of 175 'instructions' for the texts of the authors listed above.[75] The major concern of the censors is superstition (118 instructions, i.e. 67.4%). In this category, we find Laguna (50 instructions), the *Thesaurus* in Latin (36) and Spanish (5), Cabreira (8) and Rueus (19). In three cases, the texts are in the vernacular (Laguna and *Tesoro de pobres* in Spanish, Cabreira in Portuguese). With the case of Laguna at hand, José Pardo Tomás has pointed out the high attention paid by censors to books making classic authors available in the vernacular.[76] But it is clear that the Latinists (38% of the instructions in this category), who were mostly part of the scientific community, were not excluded from what seems to be an attack against popular medicine practised by ill-informed practitioners. Popular medicine has a rather uncertain reception, addressing both popular and learned readers. In Cabreira, two passages hinting at semi-religious and semi-medical *curandeirismo*, used among the *benzedeiros* and *saludadores*, are deleted as the anachronistic prayers in a remedy against epilepsy (*gota coral*): "Take pennyroyal and give it to drink with wine saying the Pater noster and Ave Maria, it is from Dioscorides."[77] The suppression was not made for the sake of historical accuracy, but in accordance with the prohibition of sacred words for profane purpose.[78]

---

75 Number of instructions by the author: Amato Lusitano, 5 (3 in 1581, 2 in 1624); Argenterius, 1; Laguna, 57; Libavius, 9; Pietro d'Abano, 14; Rueus, 19; Rueffus, 2; Sabuco, 4; Sequeira, 1; Taurellus, 4; *Thesaurus pauperum, Tesoro de pobres* and Cabreira, 49; Zwinger, 9.

76 José Pardo Tomás, *Ciencia y censura: La Inquisición española y los libros científicos en los siglos XVI y XVII* (Madrid, 1991), 136.

77 Gonçalo Cabreira, *Compendio de muytos e varios remedios de cirugia* (Braga, 1613), 30-31: "Tomemse poejos, e demlhos a beber com vinho, 'dizendo o Pater noster, e Ave Maria,' he de Dioscorides."

78 *Index librorum prohibitorum* (Rome, 1596), B2r: "verba Scripturae sacrae, quaecumque ad profanum usum impie accommodatur."

The Portuguese launched the censorship of Laguna's translation of Dioscorides with comments. Very few Classical texts appear in the Index, like Lucian's anti-Christian writings.[79] But in this case, as the Spanish Index of 1632 explains, the book is full of divinations and superstitions (*agorerias y supersticiones*), which must be removed because the ignorant could take them for granted.[80] Nevertheless, this is less severe than the Portuguese censorship, as it omits 15 suppressions. On the 58 passages which were to be expurgated in 1624, eight are motivated by reasons other than medical superstition: paganism (3), Catholic doctrine about the Golden Age (2), and astrology (1); in one case, sixty verses on vines in Spanish (V, 1, Annotation) were eliminated; finally, on the title page, the book is dedicated to King Philip II, son of Charles V, and both were qualified as "divine" (*divus*), which was to be erased.[81] This instruction would not be reproduced in the Spanish Index of 1632.

A more detailed analysis of what would shortly be classified as superstitious would lead to the distinction between superstitions and healing remedies, the former of which are rather a matter for *obscoenae* or *lascivae*, like the plant by which young girls can recover their virginity (IV, 121, annotation). This brief comparison reveals some discrepancies between the Indexes of a sensitive nature (authors, texts, deletions) and prove that, although censorship might be a common task, the Portuguese and Spanish Inquisitions, who worked independently from each other even during the period of the double monarchy, collaborated without always working hand in hand.[82]

---

79   On the issue of the expurgation of the Classics, see Hervé Baudry, "La microcensure des classiques (XVIe-XVIIe siècles): Perspective diachronique et analyse locale d'efficacité," *Res antiquitatis*, 6 (forthcoming).

80   *Novus Index*, 1632, 63: "Para lo que se sigue, assi en el Texto de Dioscorides, como en las Anotaciones del Doctor Laguna, advierta el Lector, que aunque en los Autores profanos, Griegos, o Latinos, no se nota, ni se expurga cosa alguna, aunque tengan supersticiones o hechizerias, como gente que o tuvo luz de Evangelio: como ni tampoco se quitan las agorerias, y supersticiones de los sueños de Artemidoro; mas por el peligro que estas cosas pueden tener para el vulgo de los ignorantes, que las crean como verdaderas, o quieran usar dellas, si andan el vulgar, se deven notar, y prohibir, en qualquier lengua de las vulgares, que no sea su original, en que fueron escritas, como aqui se haze en Dioscorides buelto en romance."

81   On this literary piece, see José M. Pérez Fernández, "Andrés Laguna: Translation and the Early Modern Idea of Europe," *Translation and Literature*, 21 (2012) (<http://digibug.ugr. es/bitstream/10481/21880/1/Translation_and_the_EMod_Idea_of_Europe_Repository. pdf>, 13, last accessed April 21, 2018).

82   On the autonomy and continuity of the Portuguese Inquisition from 1581 to 1640, see Paiva and Marcocci, *História*, 133-159. On the collaboration of the Iberian Inquisitions, see

Sixteen passages which were to be deleted dealt with medical astrology, the majority of them (14) from the *Conciliator* of Pietro d'Abano, and one in Laguna and Sequeira. In Avelar's entry, which referred to the 1586 bull of Sixtus V against astrology and magic, the censors advise that astrological judgements must be read with caution in medicine, navigation and agriculture. In Sequeira, who writes on the same matter, the passage to be deleted is a sixty-verse poem on prognostication in Portuguese. Furthermore, some texts incorporate theology or natural philosophy: Sabuco and Rueffus on the soul, Argenterius on semen (namely the expression "*semen est homo*" from Aristotles).

There is also a set of expurgations with overt religious contents, in a wider sense: according to rule 10 of the Council of Trent, Libavius's *Expositio* on Arnau de Vilanova and Ramón Llull, two heretical Catalans of the Middle Ages; according to article 2 of the *Instructio* of 1596, three "pagan" propositions in Laguna's paganism (God as the unique inventor of medicine; Diana, the goddess of love; on Aristippus's sovereign good); in one of the three passages, Taurellus's indifference whether you believe in Christ or Aristotle (V, 3); two passages regarding Judaism in Amato Lusitano, one from his oath (*Centuriae*, VI and VII); and one in Rueffus regarding the cross on the monster of Ravenna.[83]

Finally, laudatory attributions are a rich source of erasures in many texts: they appear in Zwinger (8) and Libavius (3), both Protestants who praise other Protestants (hence heretics) like Johann Crato or Joachim Camerarius; and in Laguna and Taurellus (1). It is noteworthy that the *Centuriae* of Amato were particularly rich in this kind of irreverence: the Roman expurgatory of 1607 located 20 of them, and the Spanish Index of 1612, 35. The Portuguese Index of 1624 did not paginate the passages but advised that all occurrences must be removed, a task achieved in most of the copies owned by the Portuguese libraries.[84]

Conclusion

The Portuguese Inquisition was not interested in medical professionals as such, but mostly in individuals of Jewish origin. A 'long social war' was waged against people who "had to cope with the permanent threat of the Portuguese

---

François Soyer, "The Extradition Treaties of the Spanish and Portuguese Inquisitions (1500-1700)," *Estudios de historia de España*, 10 (2008), 201-238.

83   On this famous monster, see Alan Bates, *Emblematic Monsters: Unnatural Conceptions and Deformed Births in Early Modern Europe* (Amsterdam, 2005), 22-33.

84   Baudry, "Bibliographia," 28-40.

Holy Office, and more generally, with the many difficulties that derived from Catholic intolerance to their religious and cultural identity."[85] In this sense, scientific issues were secondary.[86] However, the question of Inquisitorial control on science and medicine cannot be avoided. This "all powerful bureaucracy" did have an impact on individual and collective fates.[87] Indeed, the diaspora, which has been previously discussed, can be considered a sort of brain drain, which was detrimental to the local pursuit of knowledge[88]. Many historians have argued that the Portuguese university was weakened by the anti-Judaic repression. New Christians came from a traditionally learned population in a widely illiterate country.[89] Mea has pointed out the particularly severe treatment of the literates by the Coimbra Inquisition.[90] During the sixteenth and seventeenth centuries medicine had become a 'Jewish profession' because of the high percentage of 'New Christians' in the Iberian peninsula.[91] But according to the inquisitional logic, it is not possible to be both a Jew and a Christian.[92] Accordingly, in the eyes of the inquisitors, it was not possible to be both a physician and a Jew. As Paiva has pointed out, Portugal was a country where no witch hunt (*caça às bruxas*) took place. This is literally correct, but it should be remembered that the Jews, sons of the Devil (John 8:44) and the

---

85   I borrow and translate the expression of the 'long social war' from two articles by José Veiga Torres: "Uma longa guerra social: Os ritmos da repressão inquisitorial em Portugal," *Revista de história económica e social*, 1 (1978), 55-68; "Uma longa guerra social: Novas perspectivas para o estúdio da Inquisição portuguesa – a Inquisição e Coimbra," *Revista de história de ideias*, 8 (1986), 56-70. The long citation comes from Arrizabalaga, "Garcia de Orta," 32.

86   On the early modern concept of science, see Andrew Cunningham, "The Identity of Natural Philosophy: A Response to Edward Grant," *Early Science and Medicine*, 5 (2000), 259-278.

87   "[B]urocracia omnipotente" (Révah, "Entrevista," 232). On the impact of the censorship of books on readers, see José Pardo Tomás, "Censura inquisitorial y lectura de libros científicos: Una propuesta de replanteamiento," *Tiempos modernos*, 9 (2003-2004), 1-17.

88   The concept of brain drain in the early modern context was used by Richard S. Westfall, *The Construction of Modern Science: Mechanisms and Mechanics* (Cambridge, 1971), 111.

89   Augusto da Silva Carvalho, *A Medicina portuguesa no século XVII* (Lisbon, 1940), 8; Manuel Ferreira de Mira, *História da medicina portuguesa* (Lisbon, 1947), 89-90; A. Tavares de Sousa, *Curso de história da medicina: Das origens aos fins do século XVI* (Lisbon, 1981), 438.

90   Mea, *A Inquisição*, 496.

91   David B. Rudeman, *Jewish Thought and Scientific Discovery in Early Modern Europe* (Detroit, MI, 2001), 273.

92   François Soyer, "'It is not Possible to be Both a Jew and a Christian': *Converso* Religious Identity and the Inquisitorial Trial of Custodio Nunes (1604-5)," *Mediterranean Historical Review*, 26 (2011), 81-97, 88.

Synagogue of Satan (Apocalypse 2:9) were associated with the medieval witch.[93] The Portuguese Inquisition appears to have been the most systematic hunter of Jews in early modern Europe, with the purpose of making them subjects to God's medicine.

---

93   Joshua Trachtenberg, *The Devil and the Jews* (New Haven, CT, 1943); Robert I. Moore, *The Formation of a Persecuting Society: Authority and Deviance in Western Europe 950-1250* (Malden, 2007), 33; Joel Carmichael, *The Satanizing of the Jews* (New York, NY, 1992).

Between Galen and St Paul: How Juan Huarte de San Juan Responded to Inquisitorial Censorship

Guido Giglioni
Università di Macerata
guidomaria.giglioni@unimc.it

Abstract

The *Examen de ingenios para las sciencias*, published in 1575 by the Spanish physician Juan Huarte de San Juan (1529/1530-1588), was a bold attempt to apply the principles of Galenic naturalism to a better understanding of human capabilities. Inevitably, the work also touched upon a number of theological issues, especially the delicate question of the interplay between natural abilities and supernatural gifts. When the treatise was included in the Portuguese Index of 1581, and then in the Spanish Indexes of 1583 and 1584, Huarte was allowed to amend some of his positions, as is evident in the second edition published posthumously in 1594. The aim of this article is to shed light on the identity of an 'expurgated' book by concentrating on some of the most significant changes in the *Examen* triggered by the intervention of the Spanish Inquisition. It will become apparent that Huarte's response to censorship was not acquiescence or dissembling, but active engagement with the inquisitorial challenge.

Keywords

Juan Huarte de San Juan – Galen – temperament – soul – virtue – Inquisition

"Excise the whole Chapter 7."[1] Thus ordered Cardinal Gaspar de Quiroga y Vela, Archbishop of Toledo, who from 1573 to 1594 held the position of General

---

* Università di Macerata, Dipartimento di Studi Umanistici, Via Garibaldi 20, 62100 Macerata, Italy.

1 *Index librorum expurgatorum*, ed. Gaspar de Quiroga (Madrid, 1584), f. 117v: "Capitulo septimo, quitese todo, desde el principio del titulo donde dize 'Capitulo septimo, donde se muestra que

Inquisitor of Spain, and in that capacity coordinated the work behind the Indexes of Forbidden Books, which were published in Madrid in 1583 and 1584. The book in question was the *Examen de ingenios, para las sciencias* which, as announced by the title, promised to deliver a comprehensive appraisal of all types of human skill to fit the different bodies of knowledge available at the time. The physician Juan Huarte de San Juan (1529/1530-1588) wrote the *Examen*, which was published in 1575 and soon became a very influential text. The reason why Quiroga thought that the entire chapter needed to be expunged is evident from its very title:

> Where it is shown that, although the rational soul needs the temperament of the four primary qualities to dwell in the body as well as to argue and to reason, this does not imply that that soul is perishable and mortal.[2]

---

aunque el anima racional ha menester el temperamento de las quatro calidades primeras, etc.' hasta el fin del capitulo donde dice 'Y que por esta razon apetecen estar en unos lugares, y huyen de otros sin ser corruptibles.'" I would like to thank an anonymous reader for their comments and suggestions, which helped me clarify Huarte's attempt to reconcile Galen's opinion on the human soul with the principles of Christian theology (in particular, the notion of incorporeal substances, both human and divine). Huarte argued that it was possible to explain Galen 's apparent inconsistency about the immateriality of God's substance and the materiality of the human soul by invoking Plato's 'demiurgic' function of God at the moment of the creation. In the end, as we will see, this solution did not convince the inquisitors who were examining Huarte's text.

2   Juan Huarte de San Juan, *Examen de ingenios para las ciencias*, ed. Guillermo Serés (Barcelona, 1996, henceforth "*Examen* 1996"), 215: "Donde se muestra que aunque el ánima racional ha menester el temperamento de las cuatro calidades primeras, así para estar en el cuerpo come para discurrir y raciocinar, que no por eso se infiere que es corruptible y mortal." On Huarte de San Juan, see Rafael Salillas, *Un gran inspirador de Cervantes: El doctor Juan Huarte y su Examen de ingenios* (Madrid, 1905); Mauricio de Iriarte, *El doctor Huarte de San Juan y su Examen de ingenios* (Madrid, 1948 [1938]); Carlos G. Noreña, "Juan Huarte's Naturalistic Philosophy of Man," in idem, *Studies in Spanish Renaissance Thought* (The Hague, 1975), 210-263; Jon Arrizabalaga, "Juan Huarte en la medicina de su tiempo," in Véronique Duché-Gavet, ed., *Juan Huarte au XXIᵉ siècle* (Biarritz, 2003), 65-98; Felice Gambin, *Azabache: Il dibattito sulla malinconia nella Spagna dei Secoli d'Oro* (Pisa, 2005), esp. chs. 4 and 5; idem, *Un libro che ha fatto l'Europa: L'Examen de ingenios para las ciencias di Juan Huarte de San Juan* (Verona, 2015); Rocío G. Sumillera, "Introduction," in Juan Huarte de San Juan, *The Examination of Men's Wits*, transl. Richard Carew, ed. R.G. Sumillera (London, 2014), 1-70. English translations from Huarte's *Examen* are mine.

"Temperament" here means, in characteristically medical terms, a condition of humoural balance resulting from the mixing of different, partially opposite qualities and dispositions, and it is a condition that is eminently corporeal. In itself, Huarte's statement was not necessarily unorthodox from a theological point of view. Indeed, there existed a long tradition of Galenizing Christian theology, starting with Nemesius of Emesa in the fourth century and his influential book, *De natura hominis* ("On the Nature of Man"), in which temperaments could serve crucial theological requirements (such as the sensory premises of human knowledge, the bodily functions underlying the work of virtue and freedom, the ensoulment of the foetus and the resurrection of bodies).[3] What the inqusitors found questionable in the text was a certain ambiguity and the possibility that one might interpret Huarte's position as a form of dissembled mortalism. This point had become ever more pressing after the Italian philosopher Pietro Pomponazzi (1462-1525) had demonstrated that even Aristotle could easily be charged with mortalism if one focused on the bodily side of the argument, regardless of whether the *temperamentum* was seen as a *subiectum* (an organ of life, as in Huarte) or an *obiectum* (an organ of knowledge, as in Pomponazzi).[4]

The clear-cut 'amputation' of the entire Chapter 7 prescribed by Quiroga was no small matter. That section was, in fact, one of the most important parts of Huarte's treatise; indeed, it was its backbone.[5] Could the book survive this

---

3 See Owsei Temkin, *Galenism: Rise and Decline of a Medical Philosophy* (Ithaca, NY, 1973), 81-87; Julie R. Solomon, "You've Got to Have Soul: Understanding the Passions in Early Modern Culture," in Stephen Pender and Nancy S. Struever, eds., *Rhetoric and Medicine in Early Modern Europe* (London, 2016 [2012]), 195-228; Sorana Corneanu, "Francis Bacon on the Motions of the Mind," in Guido Giglioni, James A.T. Lancaster, S. Corneanu and Dana Jalobeanu, eds., *Francis Bacon on Motion and Power* (Dordrecht, 2016), 201-229.

4 On the interplay of mortalism, physiology of knowledge and cognitive accommodation to reality, see Guido Giglioni, "Accidental Intellects: Pomponazzi on Human Imagination, Body and Mortality," in Omero Proietti and Giovanni Licata, eds., *Tradizione e illuminismo in Uriel da Costa: Fonti, temi, questioni dell'*Exame das tradiçoẽs phariseas (Macerata, 2016), 121-150.

5 It is certainly not by chance that the Roman inquisitor in charge of expurgating Huarte's *Examen* in 1605 started precisely from ch. 7, identifying at the very outset the major problems: "Nel capitolo 7 dice et benissimo che l'anima rationale è sostanza spirituale e immortale contro Galeno. Confessa ancora la scientia supernaturale et il dono di profetia car. 54. Ma dal suo discorso pare che tenga con Galeno che l'anima sia un temperamento delle quattro prime qualità elementari e che da questo temperamento depende la scientia supernaturale, et il dono di profetia." See "1605. Censura in librum *Essame degli ingegni degli huomini di Giovanni Huarte,*" in Vatican City, Archivio della Congregazione per la Dottrina della Fede (ACDF), Sant'Uffizio, *Censurae librorum 1570-1606,* n. 17, ff. 572r-572v. I would like to thank Maria Pia Donato and David Armando for providing me with a transcription of the material. On another

radical act of surgery? This is the general question I would like to address in the rest of the article. The *Examen de ingenios para las sciencias* allows us to pursue this inquiry since, in fact, the book survived Quiroga's treatment and was released posthumously in a new version edited by Huarte's son Luis Huarte in 1594.[6] Its body revealed cuts, scars and cauterizations throughout, but it also had new limbs and modified organs that allowed the book to keep functioning (and in some cases, as I will argue at the end of this article, enabled it to function better). In a way, the *Examen* of 1594 had a new physiognomy, and while this was different in several respects from that of the first edition, some of the original traits were now more distinctive and pronounced. What happened, obviously, was that Huarte had accepted the challenge and decided to raise the stakes.[7]

---

instance of censorship in 1587 involving Cardinal Bellarmine and Huarte's *Examen*, see Peter Godman, *The Saint as Censor: Robert Bellarmine between Inquisition and Index* (Leiden, 2000), 118-121.

6 On the vicissitudes related to the publication of the emended version of the *Examen* in 1594 and the resulting new inquisitorial objections, see Sumillera, "Introduction," 21-22; Leen Spruit, "Catholic Censorship of Early Modern Psychology," in Martin McLaughlin, Ingrid D. Rowland and Elisabetta Tarantino, eds., *Authority, Innovation and Early Modern Epistemology: Essays in Honour of Hilary Gatti* (Cambridge, 2015), 218-239.

7 These are the two editions in question, both published by Juan Bautista de Montoya: Juan Huarte de San Juan, *Examen de ingenios, para las sciencias. Donde se muestra la differencia de habilidades que ay en los hombres, y el genero de letras que a cada uno responde en particular. Es obra donde el que leyere con attencion hallara la maniera de su ingenio, y savra escoger la sciencia en que mas ha de aprovechar, y si por ventura la vuiere ya professado, entendera si atino a la que pedia su habilidad natural ... Va dirigida ala Magestad del Rey don Philippe nuetro señor, cuyo ingenio se declara, exemplificando las reglas y preceptos desta doctrina. Con previlegio Real de Castilla y de Aragón* (Baeza, 1575; henceforth abbreviated as "*Examen* 1575"); idem, *Examen de ingenios para las sciencias, e nel qual el lector hallara la manera de su ingenio, para escoger la sciencia en que mas a de aprovechar. Y la differencia de habilidades que ay en los hombres y el género de letras y artes que à cada uno responde en particular ... Agora nuevamente enmendado por el mismo Autor y añadidas muchas cosas curiosas y provechosas. Dirigido à la C. R. M. del Rey don Phelippe nuestro señor. Cuyo ingenio se declara, exemplificando las reglas y preceptos desta doctrina. Con nuevo previlegio del Rey N. S.* (Baeza, 1594; henceforth abbreviated as "*Examen* 1594"). It is worth pointing out that, among the various translations produced during the early modern period of the *Examen* into all major European languages, two were in English: *Examination of Men's Wits*, transl. Richard Carew (London, 1594); *Examen de Ingenios, or, The Tryal of Wits*, transl. Edward Bellamy (London, 1698). Carew's translation was, in fact, based on Camillo Camilli's Italian version of the *Examen*'s 1575 edition, and published in 1582 in Venice by Aldus Manutius. Bellamy's *Tryal of Wits*, on the other hand, was a direct translation of Huarte's 1594 expurgated edition.

In the 1575 edition, the most troubling issues of Chapter 7 were two: the assumption that the rational soul in human beings could be a perishable substance, contrary to the Christian belief in an immortal soul and to its corollary that the soul was subject to real punishments or rewards after death; and an account of the virtues as natural dispositions of the body, contrary to the Christian belief in the existence of transcendent principles of moral action originally infused by God through an act of unconditional freedom. In trying to bringing back to life his book after Quiroga's surgery, Huarte managed to re-emphasize these two crucial points. After all, the identity of the *Examen* depended on them, before and after the treatment.

Galen in Hell

Let us start our analysis of Huarte's *Examen* from the excised Chapter 7 in the 1575 edition:

> When Galen died, no doubt he went to Hell and saw by direct experience that the souls were scorched by material fire, and yet this fire could not consume or destroy them. Galen knew about the doctrine of the Gospel, but it did not accept it.[8]

This comment – so subtly suspended between the serious and the playful – can be found in a marginal note in Huarte's *Examen*. No doubt, there were a good number of Galenists at the time who, indeed, liked to play with fire.[9] Huarte's brief aside on Galen in Hell suggested that, ironically, human beings would know whether their mind was immortal or not only when they died; but it also intimated, tragically, that it was only at that point that they would be directly confronted with the question of justice and would then realize how urgent this question was. Huarte also hinted at the fact that, unlike Plato and Aristotle, Galen had had the advantage to know about the Christians and their religious practices, but he had decided that he did not need to follow their path

---

8   *Examen* 1996, 216: "En muriendo Galeno, es cierto que descendío al infierno y vio por experiencia que el fuego material quemaba a las ánimas y no las podía gastar ni consumir. Este médico tuvo noticia de la doctrina evangélica y no la recibió. Libro II *De differentia pulsus*, cap. III." See also *Examen* 1575, f. 100r. See Galen, *De differentia pulsuum*, II, 3-4, in Galen, *Opera omnia*, ed. C.G. Kühn, 20 vols. (Leipzig, 1821-1833), vol. 8, 579. On Galen's views concerning the Christians, see Richard Walzer, *Galen on Jews and Christians* (London, 1949); James A. Kelhoffer, *Conceptions of "Gospel" and Legitimacy in Early Christianity* (Tübingen, 2014), 338-341.
9   The most famous of these Galenists was certainly Michael Servetus (1509/1511-1533).

to salvation. The Greeks preferred to follow the sceptical course of reason, Galen proudly reasserted.[10] On the contrary, Huarte declared (in more prudent terms) that, since in our mortal life we are not able to demonstrate in an incontrovertible manner whether the rational soul was in fact mortal or immortal, the only safe conclusion one could draw from this dilemma was that "our faith alone gives us a certain and firm belief that this soul persists forever."[11]

In Huarte's account, therefore, Galen held a fundamentally agnostic position about the immortality of the human intellect (*entendimiento*) while acknowledging that God existed from the many traces of wisdom and providence (*sabiduría y providencia*) one could see manifested everywhere in the universe. While in the Christian tradition, the human soul as an image of God ("a most wise man who is similar to Him") shared with its creator the status of incorporeal and immortal substance, Galen, in Huarte's interpretation, had failed to demonstrate the link between the two substances.[12] Here Huarte quoted Galen's words from *Quod animi mores corporis temperamenta sequantur*, the treatise devoted to demonstrating the soul's dependence on the body, in the translation by Bartolomeo Silvani, a physician, philologist and philosopher active in the Veneto in the middle of the sixteenth century: "God was not created sometime, for He is always unbegotten and eternal."[13] To add to the ambiguity in Galen's position (bodily nature of the soul and incorporeal substance of God), in the treatise on the formation of the foetus, *De formatione foetus*, Galen had assumed that the level of sophistication involved in the process of reproduction was so high that this activity could not be simply attributed to the effects of natural heat or to the power of the human rational soul. The cause had to be something more divine (if not God Himself), an "inteligencia muy sabia." Was this *inteligencia* the human soul itself or was it God acting directly in nature every time a living being was born? For Huarte this was a clear inconsistency in Galen's argument.

---

10   Galen, *De differentia pulsuum*, 577-580.

11   *Examen* 1996, 216: "sola nuestra fe divina nos hace ciertos y firmes, que dura para siempre jamás." See *Examen* 1575, f. 100r.

12   *Examen* 1996, 218. See below, footnote 16.

13   *Examen* 1996, 217; *Examen* 1575, f. 100v. See Galen, *Quod animi mores corporis temperaturas sequantur*, XI, in Galen, *Opera quae ad nos extant omnia*, ed. Janus Cornarius (Basel, 1549), 1233B: "Deus nec factus est aliquando, cum perenniter ingenitus sit ac sempiternus." On Bartolomeo Silvani, see Giuseppe Brunati, *Dizionarietto degli uomini illustri della riviera di Salò* (Milan, 1837), 136. For a recent English translation of the *Quod animi mores*, see Galen, *The Capacities of the Soul Depend on the Mixtures of the Body*, in Galen, *Psychological Writings*, ed. P.N. Singer, with contributions by Daniel Davies and Vivian Nutton (Cambridge, 2013), 333-424.

Significantly, Huarte used Hippocrates – more specifically the Hippocratic treatise on *Airs, Waters and Places* – to expose Galen's contradiction and to produce a fascinating counter-argument based on the concept of geographical place. The place for the soul was not only the body in which it dwelt, but, in keeping with the principles of Hippocratic environmentalism, was also the physical milieu in which that particular body lived; which is the same as to say that anatomy needed to be supplemented by geography. In the *Examen*, Huartes addressed Galen directly in the second person:

> You [Galen] suspect that the rational soul is perishable because, if the brain is well tempered, it is much better suited to argue and to philosophize, and if it grows warmer or colder than it is supposed to be, then it becomes delirious and talks much nonsense. The same thing can be said about the works which you claim are made by God, for if there is a man in temperate places, where the heat does not overcome the cold, nor does moisture overcome dryness, this man comes out very ingenious and discerning, while if the region is distempered, they all turn out dull-witted and ignorant.[14]

But if that was the case, Huarte objected, then perhaps God was not the unbegotten and eternal being He had revealed Himself to be, for all that He made was exposed to change and decay.[15] Precisely because of these inconsistencies, Huarte thought that Plato's understanding of God and the creation as expounded in the *Timaeus* was more correct (*más acertado*):

> although God is eternal, omnipotent and infinitely wise, He behaves as a natural agent in his works and is subjected to the disposition of the four primary qualities, in such a way that, in order to engender a most wise man who is similar to Him, He needed to find a place that was the most tempered in the universe, where the heat of the air did not overcome the cold, nor did moisture overcome dryness. And so Plato said: "God, who

---

14   *Examen* 1996, 217: "Tú sospechas ser el ánima racional corruptible porque si el celebro está
        bien templado acierta muy bien a discurrir y filosofar, y si se calienta o enfría más de lo
        que conviene, delira y dice mil disparates. Eso mesmo se infiere considerando las obras
        que tú dices ser de Dios; porque si hace un hombre en lugares templados donde el calor
        no excede a la frialdad, ni la humidad a la sequedad, le saca muy ingenioso y discreto, y si
        es la región destemplada, todos los saca estultos y necios." See *Examen* 1575, ff. 100v-101r.
15   *Examen* 1996, 217: "Pues sospechar que Dios es corruptible porque con unas calidades
        hace bien estas obras, y con las contrarias salen erradas, no lo puede confesar Galeno,
        pues ha dicho que Dios es sempiterno." See *Examen* 1575, f. 101r.

loves beauty and wisdom, first of all chose and offered a place to be inhabited which would produce human beings who were the most similar to Him."[16]

The Timaeic God, in Huarte's account, operated with a kind of matter that was already existing, and He could only bring about the better result given the circumstances. In this type of explanation, places and organs (tools) were as important as bodies. Countering Galen, Huarte argued that the fact that mental states could be affected by the use of wine and drugs did not necessarily imply that the mind in itself was corporeal and corruptible. He provided the example of a good painter whose painting did not particularly stand out because he was forced to use a bad brush.[17] While the emphasis on the body could suggest that the soul was corporeal as well, the emphasis on places (the environment) and tools (organs) suggested that the operations of the soul (an immaterial and immortal soul) were subjected to the influence of external circumstances (be they places or tools, as in the example of the painter's brush). To strengthen his argument, Huarte added an *a fortiori* argument: if even the devil, who alledgedly was a substance that was more perfect than the rational soul, could be affected by heat (as had been proven by many testimonies past and present, biblical and contemporary) without losing the prerogative of being an immortal being, then the influence that corporeal qualities exercised on the human mind could not be used as evidence that the soul was mortal.[18] And the reason was that, "despite being the lowest of all the intelligences, the rational soul has the same nature as the devil and the angels."[19] For Huarte this was the proof that human minds, demons and angels were able to perceive the objects of the senses, to be affected by material qualities and to feel emotions such as joy and sadness.

---

16   *Examen* 1996, 218: "aunque Dios es eterno, omnipotente y de infinita sabiduría, que se ha como agente natural en sus obras y que se sujeta a la disposición de las cuatro calidades primeras, de tal manera que para engendrar un hombre sapientísimo y semejante a él, tuvo necesidad de buscar un lugar, el más templado que había en todo el mundo, donde el calor de l'aire no excediese a la frialdad, ni la humidad a la sequedad. Y, así, dijo: 'Deus vero, quasi belli et sapientiae studiosus, locum qui viros ipsi simillimos producturus esset, electum in primis incolendum praebuit'." Cf. *Examen* 1575, f. 101v. See Plato, *Timaeus*, 30D-31A.

17   *Examen* 1996, 217-219; *Examen* 1575, ff. 102r-103r.

18   *Examen* 1996, 221; *Examen* 1575, f. 104v.

19   *Examen* 1996, 221-222: "El ánima racional, puesto caso que es la más ínfima de todas las inteligencias, pero tiene la mesma naturaleza que el demonio y los ángeles." *Examen* 1575, f. 105r-v.

By combining the Timaeic concept of God with the Hippocratic notion of place, Huarte thus established a parallelism between the activity of the soul in a body and that of God within the sphere of His creation. Just as God remained the immaterial and eternal principle that happened to operate in a world of matter and material necessity, so the human soul, despite being incorporeal, acted within a world of bodies, places and objects. To corroborate this point, Huarte resorted again to the notion of Hell. This time he referred to the biblical story of Lazarus and the Rich Man. Huarte conjectured that all the doubts concerning the soul, God and the afterlife vanished in the mind of the Rich Man when he finally arrived in Hell: "All these doubts dropped in the soul of the Rich Man, about whom St Luke recounts that he looked up in Hell and saw Lazarus, who was in Abraham's bosom."[20]

Through the concept of Christian Hell, Huarte was testing ideas concerning the material dispositions of the human soul, the limits of mental consciousness and the possibility that the fundamental tenets of pagan wisdom could be reconciled with the Christian faith. In the fifteenth century Marsilio Ficino (1433-1499), in a well-known passage of his *Theologia Platonica*, had used the representational ability of the imagination to explain the relationship between the immortal mind and the perception of physical pain in hell.[21] How could our disembodied mind still be affected by the *obiecta*, the representations of reality mediated by the senses? The perception of the punishment in Hell was, as it were, imaginary and yet painful – extremely painful. Huarte followed this explanatory pattern borrowed from theological literature to confirm his thesis that the human mind could not perceive or operate in ways that did not take into consideration the presence of suitable organs, places and objects. By and large, Huarte's defence strategy, before and after the inquisitorial censures (that is, both preemptively and retroactively), was to show that his theories on the faculties of the mind had a foundation in theology and in the biblical

---

20   *Examen* 1996, 224: "Todas estas dudas soltara bien el ánima del rico avariento de quien
       cuenta San Lucas que estando en el infierno alzó los ojos y vio a Lázaro que estaba en el
       seno de Abraham." *Examen* 1575, f. 109r. See Luke 16:19-31.

21   Marsilio Ficino, *Platonic Theology* (XVIII, 10), eds. Michael J.B. Allen and James Hankins,
       with William Bowen, 6 vols. (Cambridge, MA, 2001-2006), vol. 6, 196-199. On this topic, see
       Robert Klein, "L'Enfer de Ficin," in Enrico Castelli, ed., *Umanesimo e esoterismo* (Padua,
       1960), 47-84, republished in Robert Klein, *La forme et l'intelligible* (Paris, 1970), 89-124;
       Anna Corrias, "Imagination and Memory in Marsilio Ficino's Theory of the Vehicles of the
       Soul," *The International Journal of the Platonic Tradition*, 6 (2012), 81-114. On the development
       of the notion of Hell, see Alan E. Bernstein, *The Formation of Hell: Death and Retribution
       in the Ancient and Early Christian Worlds* (Ithaca, NY, 1993). On the influence of
       Ficinian motifs in Spain, see Susan Byrne, *Ficino in Spain* (Toronto, 2015).

tradition. It was important to secure this theological and exegetical premise, for at the core of the treatise lay a radically naturalistic account of human skills, in which both knowledge and action rested on specific material conditions (places, organs and objects).

Theological underpinnings are also evident in the way in which Huarte addressed the question of the virtues. As we have just seen, in Huarte's universe, God created nature so that all human skills depended on the bodily constitution of each individual:

> Since God is the author of nature, and considering that, as I said earlier, nature gives only one difference in skill (*ingenio*) to each human being, as these differences are opposed to each other or difficult to combine, He adjusts Himself to nature and, of the sciences that He freely (*gratuitamente*) distributes among human beings, it would be extraordinary if more than one were in eminent degree.[22]

In the 1575 edition, in the 'Second Proem to the Reader,' Huarte had bolstered this particular point by using a quotation from Paul's first letter to the Corinthians (I, 12:4-11).[23] To give extra support to the thesis that specific abilities

---

22   *Examen*, 1996, 49: "Porque siendo Dios el autor de Naturaleza, y viendo que ésta no da a cada hombre más que una diferencia de ingenio, como atrás dije, por la oposición o dificultad que de juntarlas hay, se acomoda con ella; y, de la ciencias que gratuitamente reparte entre los hombres, por maravilla da más que una en grado eminente." See *Examen* 1575, f. 6r; *Examen* 1594, ff. 5v-6r. The sentence in which Huarte states that God "se acomoda con ella [i.e., nature]" is, indeed, extremely problematic from the point of view of Christian theology; less so when read in Platonic terms. Carew translated "he applied himselfe to her" (*Examination of Men's Wits*, A6v), while Bellamy went with "he accommodates himself to her" (*The Tryal of Wits*, a6r). Both ways, the odd and heterodox assumptions resulting from Huarte's reading of Hippocrates and Plato (i.e., that God adapts Himself to nature) remain.

23   I Corinthians, 12:4-11 (King James Version): "Now there are diversities of gifts, but the same Spirit. And there are differences of administrations, but the same Lord. And there are diversities of operations, but it is the same God which worketh all in all. But the manifestation of the Spirit is given to every man to profit withal. For to one is given by the Spirit the word of wisdom; to another the word of knowledge by the same Spirit; To another faith by the same Spirit; to another the gifts of healing by the same Spirit; To another the working of miracles; to another prophecy; to another discerning of spirits; to another divers kinds of tongues; to another the interpretation of tongues: But all these worketh that one and the selfsame Spirit, dividing to every man severally as he will. For as the body is one, and hath many members, and all the members of that one body, being many, are one body: so also is Christ. For by one Spirit are we all baptized into one body, whether we be

depended on specific human bodies he also quoted from the Gospel of Matthew (25:15):

> I have no doubt that God carries out this distribution of disciplines taking into account the skill (*ingenio*) and the natural disposition of each individual. For St Matthew says that the talents distributed by God had been given by Him "according to everyone's virtue" [25:15]. And to think that these supernatural sciences do not require specific dispositions in the subject before they are infused in it is a very serious mistake.[24]

Here Huarte agued that the meaning of his own medical notion of *disposicion* was the same as the one denoted by Matthew's *virtus* (δύναμις). It goes without saying that this paragraph was one of those to be expurgated in the 1594 edition. In the version published in 1575, after the comparison between *disposicion* and *virtus*, Huarte had expanded on this analogy as follows:

> It is certain that when God created Adam and Eve, before filling them with wisdom (*sabiduría*), he shaped their brain in such a way that they could receive that wisdom without difficulty and the brain could be a convenient tool for arguing and reasoning. And this is what the divine scripture says: "And He gave them the heart to think and He filled them with the discipline of the intellect."[25]

The short excerpt from the Bible is from Sirach (17:5-6), also known as the Book of Ecclesiasticus. In the *Examen* there are several passages similar to this one,

---

Jews or Gentiles, whether we be bond or free; and have been all made to drink into one Spirit. For the body is not one member, but many."

24 *Examen* 1996, 50: "Este repartimiento de ciencias yo no dudo sino que le hace Dios teniendo cuenta con el ingenio y natural disposición de cada uno. Porque los talentos que repartío por San Mateo, dice el mismo Evangelista que los dio *unicuique secundum propriam virtutem*. Y pensar que estas ciencias sobrenaturales no piden ciertas disposiciones en el sujeto antes que se infundan es error muy grande." See *Examen* 1575, f. 6r. This paragraph in the 'Second Proem to the Reader' was excised in the 1594 edition and replaced with the following words: "La razon desto es que las sciencias sobre naturales se han de subjetar en el anima racional, y qualquiera anima esta sujeta al temperamento y compostura del cuerpo, come forma substancial" (*Examen* 1594, f. 6v).

25 *Examen* 1996, 50-51: "Porque cuando Dios formó a Adán y a Eva es cierto que, primero que los llenase de sabiduría, les organizó el celebro de tal manera que la pudiesen recibir con suavidad y fuese cómodo instrumento para con ella poder discurrir y raciocinar. Y así lo dice la divina Escritura: 'Et cor dedit illis excogitandi, et disciplina intellectus replevit illos.'" See *Examen* 1575, ff. 5v-7r; *Examen* 1594, f. 6v.

where Huarte is at pains to demonstrate that the letter of the Bible can be reconciled with anatomical evidence. Huarte seems not to be particularly perplexed that what for a Galenist like him is the brain the Bible describes as the heart. The essential point for Huarte is to demonstrate that the functioning of a faculty requires the appropriate organ. In a marginal note, he quotes Cicero's subtle discussion of the relationship betweek *ingenium, fortuna* and *natura* from *De officiis*.[26] This paragraph in the *Examen* is, indeed, an interesting blend of quotations and references: Sirach, Matthew, Paul and Cicero. It is in situations as exegetically complex as this that, as is often the case with the *Examen*, Huartes skilfully interweaves pagan and Christian sources to reaffirm the thesis that the adaptation of incorporeal being to material reality is a process that occurs everywhere in nature, ever since its very beginning, when God created the universe and, above all, fashioned humans out of mud.[27]

In Chapter 4 (which became Chapter 7 in the 1594 edition), referring to the case of a phrenetic woman capable of divining vices and virtues in other people, Huarte assures the reader that the phenomenon is as anatomically intelligible as the primordial wisdom (*sabiduría*) of Adam and Eve, and as the ability to discern good from evil spirits (*discretio spirituum*) described by Paul. In all these examples, Huarte intends to demonstrate that the supernatural gifts infused by God are 'adjusted' to the natural conditions of the recipient. Huarte makes his point by referring again to St Paul's First Letter to the Corinthians:

> Those who said that the ability of the phrenetic woman to detect virtues and vices in the people who went to visit her was the work of the devil should know that God gives human beings a certain kind of supernatural grace so that they may grasp and know which works come from God and which ones from the devil. St Paul includes this grace among the divine gifts and calls it *discretio spirituum*, the "discernment of the spirits," through which we know whether it is the devil or a good angel who affects us. Since the devil often comes to deceive us under the appearance of a good angel, we need this grace and supernatural gift to know whether it is him and to distinguish him from the good angel.[28]

---

26   *Examen* 1996, 45; *Examen* 1575, f. 3v; *Examen* 1594, f. 3v. See Cicero, *De officiis*, I, XXXIII, 120.

27   A similar use of medical and biblical sources, and – significantly – accompanied by references to Huarte's *Examen* can be found in Uriel da Costa (*c.* 1585-1640) and his *Exame das tradiçoẽs phariseas* (1623). See Omero Proietti, *Variazioni dacostiane: Studi sulle fonti dell'*Exame das tradiçoẽs phariseas (Macerata, 2017).

28   *Examen* 1996, 168-169: "Los que dijeron que las virtudes y vicios que descubría la frenética a las personas que la entraban a ver era artificio del demonio, sepan que Dios da a los hombres cierta gracia sobrenatural para alcanzar y conocer qué obras son de Dios y

So far so good for the inquisitors. It was the rest of the passage that did not pass the inquisitorial test and was subjected to expurgation in the 1594 edition:

> Those who have no skill for natural philosophy will be far removed from this gift (for this kind of knowledge [*ciencia*] and the supernatural one infused by God fall on one same power [*potencia*], which is the intellect [*entendimiento*]), if it is true that, in distributing his graces (for the most part) God adjusts Himself to the natural good of each individual, as I said above.[29]

As in the case of Adam and Eve, and once more using St Paul as his most authoritative source, Huarte intended to demonstrate that the supernatural gifts infused by God were 'adjusted' to the natural aptitudes of the recipient. What is more, Huarte here emphasized the importance of the constitutively individual nature of the subject, a point that was crucial in both medical and theological terms, and which could be reconciled – so Huarte wishfully thought – with the age-old Galenic notion of *temperamentum* (understanding by temperament the anatomical body, the host of environmental and climatic factors impinging on human life, and the organ of knowledge active through the senses and the imagination, i.e., the brain).

The Textual Identity of an Expurgated Book: Infected Bodies of Knowledge

Today we assume that issues concerning salvation and virtue should have no place in a treatise dealing with medico-political topics such as Huarte's *Examen*. In fact, the two words *salud* and *virtud* underwent key semantic shifts of an ethico-theological nature in that treatise. Salvation and virtue are an integral part of Huarte's central argument because, firstly, the *Examen* is a book about

---

cuáles del demonio, la cual cuenta San Pablo entre los dones divinos y la llama *discretio spirituum*; con la cual se conoce si es demonio o algún ángel bueno el que nos viene a tocar. Porque muchas veces viene el demonio a engañarnos con apariencia de buen ángel, y es menester esta gracia y este don sobrenatural para conocerle y diferenciarlo del bueno." See *Examen* 1575, f. 59r-v; *Examen* 1594, f. 109r-v.

29   *Examen* 1996, 168-169: "De este don estarán más lejos los que no tienen ingenios para la filosofía natural (porque esta ciencia y la sobrenatural que Dios infunde caen sobre una mesma potencia, que es el entendimiento), si es verdad que (por la mayor parte) Dios se acomoda en repartir las gracias al buen natural de cada uno, como arriba dije." Cf. *Examen* 1575, f. 59v.

the soul, and more specifically, about that part of the soul that is the *enten-dimiento* (with all the related questions at the time on whether the intellect is mortal or immortal, 'organic' or 'inorganic'), and secondly, because the approach is avowedly practical from the very beginning: the virtues in question are both the free and unconditional gifts mentioned in the Pauline letters (faith, hope and charity) and the moral excellencies of the classical tradition (prudence, justice, temperance and fortitude); most of all, though, they are the anatomical *virtutes*, that is, the faculties resulting from specific combinations of corporeal qualities. The ambiguity is evident, and Huarte could hardly hide his intellectual commitment, sophisticated as his attempt might be. He wrote his work at a time when the control of human thinking had already assumed forms of institutional and organized action. Despite Huarte's cautions the book was, in fact, subjected to inquisitorial investigation after it was published in 1575.[30]

Rewriting a text, or parts of a text, to comply with inquisitorial expurgation orders was a complex matter, involving delicate acts of exegetic courage and intellectual imagination. It is to Huarte's credit that, despite the numerous changes, he managed to retain the text's original physiognomy. Huarte did not shy away from the central thesis of the *Examen*: specific human skills depend on specific organizations of bodily parts, especially the brain. What he expanded from one version to the other was the apparatus of theological and biblical proofs. Guillermo Serés, the most recent editor of Huarte's *Examen*, has carefully and masterfully reconstructed all the different types of change that were introduced between the first and the second edition of the *Examen*. He distinguishes between clear-cut expunctions of questionable parts (*expurgos*), expunctions unrelated to any official demand of expurgation (*supresións aunque no por expurgo*), emendations (*enmiendas*) and additions (*adicións*).[31] To this particular grid of censored material one may add a further division into three different categories: externally induced censorship, self-censorship and voluntary change of opinion (although the boundaries between these three types of change are inevitably indistinct). We also should keep in mind that, with few exceptions, it was the 1575 edition of Huarte's book that was translated into the principal European vernaculars, which means that the allegedly heterodox

---

30   See Sumillera, "Introduction," 17-23. On medicine and the Spanish Inquisition in the early modern period, see José Pardo Tomas, *Ciencia y Censura: La Inquisición Española y los libros científicos en los siglos XVI y XVII* (Madrid, 1991), esp. 214-217.

31   See Serés's 1996 edition of Huarte's *Examen*, which I have been using throughout this article. This edition was originally published in 1989 in Madrid by Cátedra.

content of the work happened to be refracted throughout Europe by means of different languages and cultural contexts.[32]

A glance at the paratextual material of the 1575 edition shows that the book had initially been saluted as a timely and useful contribution to the improvement of social life, at all levels, from household management to civil service. The Augustinian friar Lorenzo de Villavicencio (c. 1518-1583), for instance, prefixed an 'Aprobación' that was clearly favourable to the book: "its whole doctrine is Catholic, with nothing contrary to the faith of our mother, the Holy Church of Rome." De Villavicencio, who had graduated in theology at the University of Louvain and supported Philip II's policy of involvement in the Netherlands against the Protestants, took notice of the original views championed by the author of the book (*doctrina de grande y nuevo ingenio*), based on "the best philosophy that can be taught" and with a particularly sophisticated knowledge of complex biblical loci (*toca algunos lugares de Escritura muy grave y eruditamente declarados*). Above all, De Villavicencio pointed out the social and political significance of the treatise:

> All heads of household should take the principal topic of this treatise seriously into consideration, for, if they follow what this book suggests, the Church, the state and the families will produce excellent ministers and most distinguished subjects.[33]

Antonio de Eraso, the Secretary to the Council of the Indies, signed the *licencia* for the 1575 edition on behalf of Philip II, describing the book as a remarkable achievement in which the author showed "the difference of skills (*la diferencia de habilidades*)" among human beings and the kind of discipline that was specifically required by each of them in order to blossom (*el género de letras que a cada uno responden en particular*).[34] One "doctor Heredia," signing the "Apro-

---

32   For a discussion of the main differences between the 1575 and 1594 editions, I refer the reader to Guillermo Serés, "Introducción," in Huarte de San Juan, *Examen de ingenios*, ed. G. Serés (Madrid, 1989), 13-131, at 47-71.

33   Lorenzo de Villavicencio, "Aprobación," in *Examen* 1996, 29: "He visto este libro, y su doctrina toda es católica, sin cosa que sea contraria a la fe de nuestra madre la santa Iglesia de Roma. Sin esto, es doctrina de grande y nuevo ingenio, fundada y sacada de la mejor filosofía que puede enseñarse. Toca algunos lugares de Escritura muy grave y eruditamente declarados. Su principal argumento es tan necesario de considerar de todos los padres de familia, que si siguiesen lo que este libro advierte, la Iglesia, la república y las familias ternían singulares ministros y sujetos ímportantísimos." See also *Examen* 1575, A2r; *Examen* 1594, ¶ 2r.

34   Antonio de Eraso, "Licencia, para Castilla, de la edición de 1575," in *Examen* 1996, 30: "*Examen de ingenios para las ciencias*, donde se muestra la diferencia de habilidades que

bación del Consejo de Aragón," described the author of the book as gifted with a uniquely creative mind (*singular ingenio inventivo*) and expertise in natural philosophy (*ejercitado en sutil filosofía natural*). Like De Villavicencio, Heredia praised the book for its "important usefulness for the state."[35]

And yet the *licencia* and the *aprobaciónes* did not prevent the *Examen* from becoming a target of the Inquisition. The controversial points were numerous and complex – not just those about the temperaments and virtues I have examined in this article. Unsurprisingly, the troubles had begun soon after the publication of the first edition, in 1579, when the theologian Alonso Pretel, of the Holy Office of Baeza, denounced Huarte's treatise before the Inquisition of Córdoba.[36] The *Examen* was first mentioned without the name of its author in the Portuguese Index of prohibited books of 1581, the *Catalogo dos livros que se prohibem nestes Regnos e Senhorios de Portugal*.[37] In 1583, the "Examen de ingenios, compuesto por el doctor Iuan Huarte de sant Iuan" was included in the Spanish Index, in the section devoted to "libros que se prohiben en Romance." The accompanying asterisk identified the book as one of those that could be published once they had been cleansed of their mistaken views: "no se emendando y corrigiendo."[38] A meticulous list of instructions on how to change and cut Huarte's text appeared in the *Index librorum expurgatorum* published in 1584 by Gaspar de Quiroga.[39]

When reading prefatory letters, introductions and directions prefixed to indexes of forbidden books and expurgatory catalogues, we get the clear impression that the ecclesiastic authorities were looking at the printing of books as part of the final blow that Satan and his minions were about to strike against

---

hay en los hombres y el género de letras que a cada uno responden en particular." Cf. *Examen* 1575, A3r-v.

35   Heredia, "Aprobación del Consejo de Aragón," in *Examen* 1996, 32: "Paréceme obra católica, en que el autor muestra singular ingenio inventivo, y ejercitado en sutil filosofía natural. Su argumento es exquisito entre todos los que yo he visto y oído en su género. Y, si se probase, sería sin duda de importante utilidad a la república. Tengo por provechoso el haberlo reducido a tales términos, que los ingenios puedan ejercitarse, y descubrir algunos secretos naturales, de los que el autor ofrece." Cf. *Examen* 1575, A4r-v.

36   Sumillera, "Introduction," 19; Noreña, "Juan Huarte's Naturalistic Philosophy of Man," 240. See also J.M. de Bujanda (editor in chief), *Index des livres interdits*, 11 vols. (Sherbrooke, Geneva and Montréal, 1984-2002), vol. 6 (*Index de l'Inquisition Espagnole*, 1993), 818; vol. 9 (*Index de Rome, 1596*, 1994), 372; vol. 10 (*Thesaurus de la littérature interdite au XVIe siècle*, 1996), 556.

37   Jorge de Almeida and Bartolomeu Ferreira, eds., *Catalogo dos livros que se prohibem nestes regnos e senhorios de Portugal* (Lisbon, 1581), f. 19r.

38   Gaspar de Quiroga, ed., *Index et catalogus librorum prohibitorum* (Madrid, 1583), f. 31r.

39   *Index librorum expurgatorum*, ff. 116r-118v.

an increasingly weakening Christendom. One of the reasons, the inquisitors assumed, was that the devil was taking advantage of the latest technological resources, using the mechanical reproduction of ideas to spread the poison of heresy through printed texts. Books therefore needed to be evaluated, correct-ed, edited, cut and rewritten. In other words, they needed to be cured and san-itized. The situation was one of dramatic urgency. As the censoring team supervised by Archbishop Quiroga explained in their letter opening the 1584 *Index*, the *catalogus expurgatorius* was not intended to cauterize all the infect-ed books of which they were aware, but to provide cautionary examples to be used when reading and censoring books:

> The books indicated by the catalogue of prohibitions have been expur-gated by men of proven faith and knowledge, apart from a few books (not many) for which it was not even necessary for us to provide a justifica-tion. And we decided to do so, not because they were not numerous and important, but because through the work which we are now undertaking we do not put an end to the process of emendation, but we rather set a starting point and a model. In this way, the Office of the Holy Inquisition strongly hopes that it will be then helped by the work of learned and pious men, for many more books to be expurgated are still there and will keep appearing, either because heretics never stop perverting and infect-ing all the best authors, or because some of the writings by the heretics themselves are tolerated – provided that religion is made safe – for the sake of learning. Of these works, in order to be safely handled by eve-rone's hands, some parts must necessarily and constanly be destroyed and amputated.[40]

Judging from the expurgatory instructions in the *Index* of 1584, one might say that inquisitorial control of published material was fundamentally an

---

40   "Letter to the Reader," in *Index librorum expurgatorum*, sig. **5r-v: "Expurgati sunt ab spectatae fidei et doctrinae viris libri illi quos catalogus prohibitionum designat, praeter paucos admodum quorum, cum copia non esset, ne rationem quidem haberi fuit necesse. Non tam quod neque plures, neque maioris essent momenti, quam quod hoc labore qui nunc susceptus est non est emendandi finis factus, sed initium potius et specimen datum. In quo se posthac doctorum et piorum virorum opera et studio iuvari sanctae Inquisitio-nis Officium vehementer exoptat. Restabunt enim occurrentque expurgandi multo plures, vel quia optimos quosque autores depravare et inficere haeretici nunquam desis-tent, vel quia ex catalogi regulis ipsorum quoque haereticorum scripta quaedam, quate-nus salva religione liceat, eruditionis gratia tolerantur. Ex quibus ut omnium manibus tractari tuto possint, erunt continenter aliqua necessario delenda atque amputanda."

operation of book surgery: it consisted of carrying out mental amputations and applying prosthetic thoughts. As a result, books were inevitably disfigured by the treatment. Some of them, however, responded to the intervention and came out of the experience in a different way, not necessarily emasculated, crippled or mutilated. The history of the *Examen* from 1579 to 1594 is one such story of both re-adaptation to inflicted change, and of preservation – up to a point – of the original spontaneity of the thinking act.

As Hervé Baudry also notes in this volume, it is not simply ironic or accidental that the language used by the censors was distinctively medical: the process of 'evacuation,' *expurgatio*, belonged to one of the fundamental ways followed by human beings in order to keep their body healthy – the so-called six non-naturals.[41] Likewise, to keep the body of Christendom healthy and the minds of the faithful sane there were healthy ways to regularize the ingestion of knowldge. The more food for thought one was absorbing (and thanks to the printing press individuals were, indeed, ingesting vast amounts of new information), the greater care was required to flush out heterodox toxins from the system, and thus to avoid the risk of either poisoning or spreading contagion among reading communities.

The textual identity of an expurgated book thus sheds invaluable light on the thinking process affecting minds under inquisitorial pressure. While in this present volume, Hannah Marcus investigates the behaviour of those authors who accepted this pressure and turned themselves into censors, here I have focused on the response by someone who resisted this kind of action. How do individuals who are forced to rethink themselves and their worlds respond to this most violent and unnatural act? The possibilities are many, from acquiescence to opposition (and often death), from dissimulation to simulation. Huarte belongs to a particular strand within the various types of responses enacted by a large number of early modern minds who were put under investigation by religious and political institutions. Like other sixteenth-century authors (I am thinking here of Bernardino Telesio, Girolamo Cardano and Tommaso Campanella), Huarte preferred to raise the stakes, turning oppression into intellectual challenge.[42] For him, to defend the inner logic of the argument was essential in order to preserve the original spontaneity of the thinking activity.

---

41   On the six non-naturals in the early modern period, see Sandra Cavallo and Tessa Storey, *Healthy Living in Late Renaissance Italy* (Oxford, 2013); Guido Giglioni, "I sei non-naturali nella medicina del Rinascimento," *Giornale della Accademia di Medicina di Torino*, 177 (2014) [2016], 337-348.

42   A classical study on this specific topic is Luigi Firpo, "Filosofia italiana e Controriforma," *Rivista di filosofia*, 41 (1950), 150-173; 390-401; 42 (1951), 30-47. For a more recent

Conclusion

In 1594, about twenty years after the *editio princeps*, Luis de Salazar, a civil servant of Philip II, signed the royal privilege for the emended edition of the *Examen*, which he addressed to Juan Huarte's son, Luis. The tone was still highly appreciative, but there were references to the requests by the Holy Office of the Inquisition. De Salazar noted "the great work" that Huarte had done "to correct and to complete the treatise," and that "the corrections were in accordance with the order of the last catalogue published by the members of the Council of the Inquisition." Now that Huarte had addressed all the queries raised by the inquisitors, the book could be read again as a source of ingenuity and public wisdom (*libro de mucho ingenio, útil y provechoso a la república*).[43]

Provecho was, indeed, the dominant note of the treatise: to assess the minds of human beings in order to find the right fit between aptitudes and careers. Today Huarte would sit comfortably in one of those meetings where students and instructors discuss together the importance of professionalization, specialization and employability. Conventional wisdom has it that studying is for a job, and a job is based on specific training. Huarte wrote an immensely popular treatise addressing this problem, presenting it as a matter of anatomy, pedagogy and politics at once. He was adamant that the training of skills in the young had to be mono-functional, non transferable and rigorously intradisciplinary:

---

assessment, see Saverio Ricci, *Inquisitori, censori, filosofi sullo scenario della Controriforma* (Rome, 2008). On Telesio's predicament, see Guido Giglioni, "Introduzione," in Bernardino Telesio, *De rerum natura iuxta propria principia libri IX* (Rome, 2013), pp. XI-XXXII. On Cardano's problems with the Inquisition, see Ugo Baldini, "Cardano negli archivi dell'Inquisizione e dell'Indice: Note su una ricerca," *Rivista di storia della filosofia*, 53 (1998), 761-766; Baldini and Leen Spruit, "Cardano e Aldrovandi nelle lettere del Sant'Uffizio Romano all'inquisitore di Bologna (1571-1573)," *Bruniana et Campanelliana*, 6 (2000), 145-163. On Campanella and his rewriting of the *Atheismus triumphatus* under inquisitorial pressure, see Germana Ernst, "Introduzione: Storia di un testo," in Tommaso Campanella, *L'ateismo trionfato*, ed. G. Ernst, 2 vols. (Pisa, 2004), vol. 1, VII-LV.

43 Luis de Salazar, "Privilegio para la edición de 1594," in *Examen* 1996, 37: "Por cuanto por parte de vos, Luis Huarte de San Juan, hijo legítimo del doctor Juan Huarte de San Juan, natural de la villa de San Juan del Pie del Puerto (ya difuncto) nos ha sido fecha relación: que el dicho doctor, vuestro padre, había compuesto y ordenado un libro intitulado *Examen de ingenios*, el cual había sido impreso una vez y visto por el Santo Oficio, y con algunas enmiendas que había hecho había mandado que anduviese, y al presente no se hallaba ninguno y era pedido de mucha gente; y por ser libro de mucho ingenio, útil y provechoso a la república, nos suplicastes os mandásemos dar licencia para le poder imprimir, atento el mucho trabajo que el dicho vuestro padre había pasado en enmendallo y ponello en la perfección que ahora le presentábades." Cf. *Examen* 1594, ¶3r-¶5r.

if you are a soldier you cannot be a poet, if you are a theologian you cannot be a politician. Surprising as this may sound at first, this point of view could count on Platonic support. In *The Republic*, Plato had dismissed any notion of multifunctionality among the citizens of his ideal state as both stultifying and hazardous, for the citizens, especially the so-called 'custodians,' were not supposed to be distracted from their specific tasks. A healthy state could only benefit from the cooperation between individuals with different aptitudes, according to the principle that "it is impossible for one person to carry out many skilled tasks well" (*Republic*, 370AC, 374A, 424D).[44]

The reader may have already noted a certain favourable disposition towards Plato's philosophy in Huarte's book, especially towards the cosmological and theological settings outlined in the *Timaeus*. This should not come as too much of a surprise, though. As a fervent Galenist, Huarte was, in fact, developing theoretical and practical guidelines that could revive the original medico-political inspiration behind Galen's anatomical research programme – to paraphrase a celebrated Latin proverb: *medicina sana in civitate sana*, a healthy medicine in a healthy body politic.[45] This was a research programme that intended to reconcile Hippocrates with Plato, *paideia* with medicalization. But perhaps Huarte was also using Plato to reconcile Christian faith with pagan *sabiduría* – the wisdom of Democritus, Hippocrates and Socrates, that is to say, afterlife salvation with natural adaptation, Grace with virtues. God could then be seen as a 'demiurgic' creator, who dealt with matter when fashioning the world and who adapted the soul to the material universe of the creation. Furthermore, a model of 'Timaeic' creation could also reconcile an 'anatomical' notion of virtue as *ingenio* with the Pauline notion of supernatural talent.

In the most critical chapter of his book, Chapter 7 of the 1575 edition, in which the exercise of the mental faculties was described as depending on the anatomical configuration of the body, Huarte decided to resort to biblical exegesis more than to traditional philosophical and medical arguments to show that his position could be compatible with Judeo-Christian views on the soul and its afterlife. As in the case for other authors who had been subjected to inquisitorial investigations at the time (Telesio, Cardano and Campanella), Huarte decided not to cave in to the demands of the ecclesiastic prosecutors, but to preserve a certain degree of critical autonomy and to raise the stakes of the ongoing debate. His intention was to show that, even when positing the existence of the devil and accepting the veracity of biblical parables, he was

---

44   Plato, *Republic*, eds. Chris Emlyn-Jones and William Preddy, 2 vols. (Cambridge, MA, 2013), vol. 1, 165, 180-183, 355.

45   See Galen, *The Capacities of the Soul*, 400-404.

still able to demonstrate that what he had originally stated was correct. In order to be effective in the life of individual human beings, the supernatural gifts of Grace and the eternal joys and pains after the death of the body had to be engrafted onto the particular disposition of an individual, whether this disposition was the bodily complexion (*temperamentum*), the particular geographic region (*locum*) or, on a more abstract level, the representation of reality (*phantasma* or *obiectum*).

And so Huarte imagined that when Galen descended to Hell (for he was supposed to go to Hell anyway), he had an experience similar to that of the rich man in the parable from the Gospel of Luke. He felt the pain of fire despite being an immaterial substance. It was certainly the most oxymoronic and puzzling experience he could have as a Greek doctor and a gentile. At that point, so Huarte imagined, Galen must have realized that his doctrine of the bodily temperament was compatible with the eternal life of a disembodied self – which for him meant that those Christians were right after all. Was this a *boutade* or a preemptive measure to secure the approval of the Church and to spare himself the flames of the earthly punishment? As I said at the beginning of my article, authors like Huarte were, indeed, playing with fire, and yet they continued to be intellectually stimulated by the possibility that the eternal fire was real and by the challenge of providing a plausible explanation of that fire, theologically (divine justice), philosophically (the nature of consciousness) and anatomically (perception of pain). This intellectual exercise, imposed on the minds of all kinds of savants and practioners during the early modern period, was often taken as an extraordinarily serious business by those who accepted to play this riskiest of games all the way through. This was no longer playing with the idea of a double truth (by simulating or dissimulating); this was playing with the idea that one truth, when it was presented as sufficiently inclusive, could unite rather than divide minds.[46]

---

46   Here it is worth pointing out that, despite Huarte's efforts, his *Examen*, both in the original and in its seventeenth-century translations, remained on the Roman Index until 1966, when the Index was 'suspended' by Pope Paul VI. See Julián Velarde Lombraña, "Huarte de San Juan, patrono de psicología," *Psicothema*, 5 (1993), 451-458, 452.

Medical Martyrs: Nineteenth-Century Representations of Early Modern Inquisitorial Persecution of Spanish Physicians

Andrew Keitt
University of Alabama at Birmingham
*akeitt@uab.edu**

Abstract

This essay examines the discourse on medicine and the Inquisition in nineteenth-century Spain. It traces how liberal reformers selectively appropriated aspects of the history of Spanish medicine in the service of their contemporary political and scientific agendas, and how in doing so they contributed to the formation of new professional and national identities.

Keywords

nineteenth-century history of medicine – Spanish nationalism – Inquisition – Juan Huarte de San Juan

Modern research on the Spanish Inquisition has been, in large part, a reaction to the mythologizing of the institution over the course of the nineteenth century. The French invasion of the peninsula was the catalyst for this myth-making; when the Inquisition was suppressed in 1808 at the hands of Joseph Bonaparte, who had been installed on the Spanish throne by his brother, it brought into the spotlight an institution that had been moribund for well over a century. But as Spain lurched between absolute monarchy, constitutional monarchy, and republicanism, the fate of the Inquisition came to be seen as a referendum on the kind of nation Spain was ultimately to become.[1]

---

* Department of History, 1401 University Blvd. HHB 360H Birmingham, AL 35294-1152, USA.
1 See Stephen Haliczer, "Inquisition Myth and Inquisition History: The Abolition of the Holy

During the decades following the Napoleonic Wars, the status of the Inquisition remained a political issue as conservatives championed its restoration (succeeding in 1814) and liberals its ultimate demise (succeeding provisionally in 1823, and definitively in 1834). What liberals and conservatives had in common, despite their ideological differences, was a tendency to exaggerate the Inquisition's influence; each faction portrayed the Holy Office as a formidable historical force, capable of either ensuring Spain's greatness or guaranteeing her decline.[2] These exaggerations have often been blamed for impeding an objective understanding of the Spanish Inquisition, and in response to such complaints the post-Franco historiography has made great strides in dispelling such caricatures – at least among historians, if not in the popular imagination. But the nineteenth-century myths surrounding the Inquisition can be instructive in their own right, as they have the potential to provide insight into the development of new political cultures in post-revolutionary Spain. In particular, the relationship between medicine and the Inquisition merits our attention because physicians, according to the liberal master narrative, were the quintessential victims of an oppressive, reactionary old regime that stifled free thought, political progress, and scientific advancement.[3]

Spanish physicians were politically active in the early nineteenth century in the aftermath of the Cortes of Cádiz, which had drafted Spain's first constitution. They played important roles in the public sphere and in the legislature during the establishment of a new, and precarious, liberal order.[4] This was not unusual; physicians played similar roles elsewhere in Europe and abroad.[5]

Office and the Development of Spanish Political Ideology," in Angel Alcalá, ed., *The Spanish Inquisition and the Inquisitorial Mind* (New York, NY, 1987), 523-546.

2   Ibid., 524.

3   Polemics on the relationship between the Spanish Inquisition and Spanish science have a long history, with repercussions extending into present-day scholarship. See Víctor Navarro Brotons, "La polémica sobre la Inquisición y la ciencia en la España moderna: Consideraciones historiográficas y estado actual de la cuestión," in Ugo Baldini, ed., *La polemica europea sull'Inquisizione* (Rome, 2015), 123-144.

4   Francisco Guerra, introduction to [Antonio Hernández Morejón], *Historia bibliográfica de la medicina española, obra póstuma de Don Antonio Hernández Morejón*, vol. 1 (New York, NY, 1967), vii.

5   Warwick Anderson and Hans Pols, "Scientific Patriotism: Medical Science and National Self-Fashioning in Southeast Asia," *Comparative Studies in Society and History*, 54 (2012), 93-113, on 98-99. Anderson and Pols provide as examples Rudolf Virchow, the German pathologist who took part in the revolutions of 1848, and his protégé, José Rizal, the Filipino independence leader.

Medicine wielded a great deal of cultural authority, combining as it did the twin Enlightenment ideals of scientific rationalism and practical reform, a combination that appealed to the middle class professionals who made up the vanguard of liberal nationalist movements. Medical discourse also provided, as we shall see, a rich source of metaphors for the diagnosis and treatment of the body politic.[6]

An important forum for political activism on the part of physicians in Spain was the medical press, which comprised a vast array of publications, offering content ranging from advertisements for vacant medical posts and articles on recent scientific discoveries, to book reviews, historical vignettes, commentary on current events, and political polemics. One such periodical was *El Crisol* (*The Crucible*), which in 1855 published a treatise entitled *Médicos perseguidos por la Inquisición española* ("Physicians Persecuted by the Spanish Inquisition").[7] The treatise was written under the pseudonym, "el doctor Palomeque," in reference to the famous innkeeper in Cervantes' *Don Quijote*, but the actual author was Ildefonso Martínez y Fernández, a physician and liberal reformer. In the text, Martínez unleashed a scathing indictment of the repression of medical practitioners, and medical knowledge, by the Inquisition.

These sorts of critiques were common among Spanish liberals of the period; not surprisingly, Martínez drew on Antonio Llorente's *Historia crítica de la Inquisición en España* (*A Critical History of the Inquisition of Spain*), which contained a similar inventory of inquisitorial misdeeds.[8] But what is particularly interesting from a historian's perspective is how Martínez and his peers appropriated early modern medical discourse for the purposes of their own nineteenth-century political project. Here we have an instance of liberal mythmaking that deployed the history of early modern medicine as a critique of inquisition, throne, and altar, and in so doing exemplified the complex and

---

6 Warwick and Pols, "Scientific Patriotism," 93, point to the symbolic linkages between medical science and nationalism in colonial independence movements, wherein scientifically trained political activists were able to present themselves as "modern, progressive, and cosmopolitan" in equal measure to their colonial oppressors. Spain is an interesting case in this context, as it was, on the one hand, a colonial power (however tenuously), and on the other, a scientifically backward – and perhaps not entirely European – regime in the eyes of its European rivals, and quite often in self-critical Spanish eyes as well. So José Rizal might travel from Manila to the metropole of Madrid to receive his medical training while Spanish physicians, in turn, looked to Paris and Berlin as examples of medical establishments to be emulated.

7 El Doctor Palomeque [Ildefonso Martínez y Fernández], *Médicos perseguidos por la Inquisición española* (Madrid, 1855).

8 Juan Antonio Llorente, *Historia crítica de la Inquisición de España* (Madrid, 1822).

often tendentious uses of the past in attempts to form a new Spanish national identity.[9]

A great deal has been written on how such creative uses of the past helped construct the "imagined communities" of nationalist lore, but what has gone largely unexamined, according to Warwick Anderson and Hans Pols, is the "biological character and scope of nationalism."[10] While Anderson and Pols are undoubtedly correct in their assessment of the scholarly literature on nationalism, there has, in fact, been work done on "medical politics" in early modern Spain, and the case of Ildefonso Martínez y Fernández may help illuminate the connections between this earlier tradition and the medical/biological aspects of nationalism in the nineteenth century.

Ildefonso Martínez y Fernández's treatise on physicians who ran afoul of the Inquisition was just one small part of a voluminous scientific and literary output; he wrote on physiology, epidemiology, mental illness, philosophy, literature, history, and many other topics.[11] At a young age Martínez befriended the celebrated bibliophile, Don Bartolomé José Gallardo, who encouraged him in his literary pursuits and contributed some of the documents used by Martínez in his treatise on the Inquisition. Martínez's wide-ranging intellectual interests, and his collaboration with literary figures like Gallardo, are reminiscent of the medical humanists of the sixteenth century, who inspired Martínez with their contributions to both the field of medicine and the republic of letters.[12]

---

9   In the past little was written on nationalism in Spain, perhaps because the very idea of a
     Spanish nationalism was often dismissed by historians as unworthy of study, since Spain's
     trajectory was so different from classic cases such as England, France, and Germany. In
     recent years, however, scholars have begun to fill this lacuna, although much work
     remains to be done. For a summary of some of this scholarship and a full-throated defense
     of Spanish nationalism as an object of study, see the prologue to José Álvarez Junco, *Mater
     dolorosa: La idea de España en el siglo XIX*, 14th ed. (Madrid, 2016), 11-28.

10   According to Warwick and Pols, "Scientific Patriotism," 95, "neither [Hans] Gellner nor
     Benedict Anderson critically interrogates the biological character and scope of nationalism. They emphasize the importance of education, bureaucratization, and communication in the humanistic imagining of the nation, but the specific role of science in these
     modern processes receives scant attention." See Ernest Gellner, *Nations and Nationalism*
     (Ithaca, NY, 1983) and Benedict Anderson, *Imagined Communities: Reflections on the Origin and Spread of Nationalism* (London, 1991).

11   An inventory of Martínez's works has been compiled by Mercedes Cabello Martín. See "El
     archivo personal de Ildefonso Martínez y Fernández en la Biblioteca Histórica de la Universidad Complutense de Madrid," BH AP 4.

12   On medical humanism, see Nancy G. Siraisi, *History, Medicine, and the Traditions of
     Renaissance Learning* (Ann Arbor, MI, 2007).

Martínez belonged to the first of what José María López Piñero has called the "intermediate generations."[13] This cohort was made up of liberal scientists and physicians born around the year 1820 (Martínez was born in 1821), who were responsible for beginning the restoration of Spanish science, which had undergone a precipitous decline as a result of the revolutionary upheavals of the early the nineteenth century.[14] It was left to the second intermediate generation, born around 1835, to institutionalize these gains, thereby preparing the way for a "silver age" of scientific production in Spain that took place during the first third of the twentieth century.[15] In Piñero's treatment, these two generations together were part of a broader "intermediate stage" in the history of modern Spanish medicine, and a hallmark of this stage was the formation of various medical associations that functioned simultaneously as professional lobbying groups, scientific societies, and political clubs.[16] These associations had a liberal bent, as opposed to the more conservative academies that had previously been the most common form of medical organization.[17] Typical of this new type of institution was La Sociedad Médico-Quirúgica de Emulación e Instrucción Recíproca (The Medico-Surgical Society for Emulation and Reciprocal Instruction) of which Martínez was a founding member.

While liberal physicians as a group benefitted from the end of absolutism in Spain after the death of Ferdinand VII in 1833, fissures within Spanish liberalism came to the fore during the 'moderate decade' of 1844-54 under the new constitutional monarchy of Isabel II, and these fissures were reflected within the medical profession. The moderate decade, as its name suggests,

---

13   See José María López Piñero, "Juan Bautista Peset y Vidal y las 'generaciones intermedias' del XIX español," *Medicina Española*, 46 (1961), 186-203.

14   Antonio M. Rey González, "Clásicos de la psiquiatría del siglo XIX (IX): Juan Bautista Peset y Vidal (1821-1885)," *Revista de la Asociación Española de Neuropsiquiatría*, 5, no. 12 (1985), 87-98, on 89. When it comes to Spanish science, discussions of "decline" and "restoration" are inevitably fraught. See Víctor Navarro Brotons and William Eamon, "Spain and the Scientific Revolution: Historiographical Questions and Conjectures," in Víctor Navarro Brotons and William Eamon, eds., *Más allá de la leyenda negra: España y la revolución científica* (Valencia, 2007), 27-38.

15   Ibid. On the "edad de plata," see Eduardo Hernández-Pacheco y Estevan *et al.*, *La edad de plata de la cultura española (1898-1936): Letras, ciencia, arte, sociedad y culturas*, 3rd ed., vol. 2, *Historia de España* 39 (Madrid, 1999).

16   On this intermediate stage, see José María López Piñero, "Las ciencias médicas en la España del siglo XIX," in José María López Piñero, ed., *La ciencia en la España del siglo XIX* (Madrid, 1992), 217-227. For more on these associations, see Agustín Albarracín Teulón, "Las asociaciones médicas en la España del siglo XIX," *Cuadernos de historia de la medicina española*, 10 (1971), 119-186.

17   López Piñero, "Las ciencias médicas," 219-220.

was dominated by the *moderados*, well established, elite men of property who had gained financially and professionally under the new regime and sought to steer the government of Spain toward their own private interests. The progressives, or *progresistas,* in contrast, had less of a stake in the status quo, and pursued a more radical agenda, which emphasized redistributing property and expanding the franchise. Within the medical profession, this ideological divide played out in scientific terms, with *moderado* physicians tending toward older, vitalist theories, and *progresistas* championing mechanism, positivism, and experimentalism.[18] Martínez's career reflected these divisions: As a political commentator and man of letters, Martínez penned tributes to the radical revolutionary and *progresista* hero, Rafael de Riego, wrote treatises celebrating participatory democracy and popular sovereignty, and advocated for "universal emancipation" from societies that promoted the "exaltation of the few and the brutalization of the masses."[19] As a physician, he was skeptical of vitalism, exhorting his fellow physicians as follows:

> Fanatical mortals, stop enquiring after first causes and essences – study only the effects; observe, experiment, interrogate nature with modesty, and thus shall you advance your investigations! In effect, gentlemen, have we advanced physiology more with the invention of a 'vital principle' and the deliriums of Paracelsus than through the observation and practice of Galen and Hippocrates? Certainly not; rather we have set back our knowledge of effects that are clearly due to alterations in the organization [of the body], attributing them instead to this particular principle, which is sometimes considered a form of intelligence, and other times no, and which serves above all to manifest our insufficiency. We use the word as if it meant that we actually know something, but in resorting to this explanation we only prove our own ignorance [...]. The word 'vital' is how we doctors describe something that we do not understand, like the physicists with their 'attraction,' and the chemists with their 'affinity.'[20]

---

18   Ibid., 218.

19   "Discurso pronunciado por D. Ildefonso Martínez en el aniversario de la muerte de D. Rafael del Riego (n.d.)," BH AP 4, leg. 3, Nº 3; "La democracia o el porvenir (n.d.)," BH AP 4, leg. 3, Nº 5; "Proyecto de una emancipación universal (1847)," BH AP 4, leg. 3, Nº 4.

20   "¡Fanaticos mortales, dejad de inquirir las causas primitivas, esenciales, estudiad solo los efectos, observad, experimentad, interrogad con modestia a la naturaleza, y adelantereís en vuestras investigaciones! En efecto Señores ¿hemos adelantado nosotros mas la fisiologia, con la invencion del principio vital y los devaneos del Paracelso que con la observacion y practica de un Galeno y un Hipocrates? Ciertamente que no; antes bien hemos retardado los conocimientos y efectos debidos á alteraciones manifiestas en la

Martínez also took a keen interest in contemporary debates over the relationship between mind and brain; he criticized those who posited a strict separation between the two, i.e. the 'spiritualists' who saw a naturalized psychology as a threat to religion and morality. Typical of this mindset was the work of Patricio Azcárate, which portrayed materialism as an affront to the Spanish national character:

> The philosophy of the prevailing curriculum, lacking in elevation and dignity, is that of materialism; and once science has been materialized I do not know how society can avoid becoming materialized as well. And the Spaniard, who is instinctively a spiritualist due to his race, his elevated sentiments, and his religious beliefs, how will he avoid being contaminated by these empirical tendencies and denaturing his character?[21]

Against this backdrop, attempts to explain character traits in terms of brain functions, as in the increasingly popular phrenological researches of Gall and Spurzheim, were seen as dangerously subversive.[22] While Martínez criticized aspects of phrenology and denied being a doctrinaire materialist himself, he shared the conviction that the brain comprised a diversity of material organs, which functioned according to the ordinary laws of nature and were ultimately responsible for cognition. He insisted that his task was to leave issues

---

organizacion, los hemos atribuido a ese principio particular que muchas veces se le considera como inteligente, y otras no, que en suma desconocemos, no valiendo mas que manifestar nuestra insuficiencia, quedando tan convencidos con la palabra como si realmente supiesemos algo envolviendo en esa esplicacion la mas completa prueba de nuestra ignorancia, siendo de advertir que la palabra vital es á donde dirijimos los facultativos, aquello que no entendemos, como los fisicos á su atraccion, y los quimicos á su afinidad." Ildefonso Martínez y Fernández, *Del influjo de lo físico en lo moral y viceversa: Discurso pronunciado en el Ateneo Médico de Madrid* (Madrid, 18 April 1842). BH AP 4, leg. 1, Nº 6. All translations mine, unless otherwise noted. I have retained the punctuation and accentuation of the original sources with some minor exceptions in the interest of clarity.

21 "La filosofía del plan de estudios vigente, sin elevación y sin dignidad, es la filosofía de la materia; y materializada la ciencia no sé cómo deje de materializarse la sociedad. Y el español, que es espiritualista por instinto, por raza, por elevación de sentimientos y por sus creencias religiosas, ¿es acreedor a que se le inocule en estas tendencias empíricas y se desnaturalice su carácter?" Patricio de Azcárate, *Veladas sobre la filosofía moderna* (Madrid, 1853), 12. Quoted in Enric J. Novella, "El discurso del yo: el espiritualismo psicológico en la cultura española de mediados del siglo XIX," *Asclepio*, 65, no. 2 (2013), 16.

22 On the contemporary controversies surrounding phrenology, see Elizabeth A. Williams, *The Physical and the Moral: Anthropology, Physiology, and Philosophical Medicine in France, 1750-1850* (Cambridge, 1994), 179.

pertaining to "the spiritual and the immortal to the theologians and focus on the facts that experience and observation yield to physicians who have occupied themselves with such matters."[23]

Turning now to Martínez's treatise itself, he begins the work with a pledge to "analyze medically" the Holy Office in order that his readers may "learn the lessons of the past," motivated by a "hatred for the executioners and tyrants of thought."[24] He then sets out, first, to record the names of the victims, and second, to relate details from the most famous trials of the Spanish Inquisition. Following this approach, Martínez summarizes the cases of celebrated physicians such as Francisco Lopez de Villalobos, the court physician to both Ferdinand of Aragon and Carlos v, who came under inquisitorial scrutiny due to his Jewish origins, and Juan de Nicholás y Sacharles, who was forced to flee Spain on account of his Protestant sympathies. Martínez concludes with a paean to his medical martyrs:

> Here's to you, O great physicians persecuted by the Inquisition: yes, here's to you, illustrious martyrs; some of you suffered imprisonment, some the San Benito, others the bonfire, but your colleagues in the sciences have freed countless victims from your oppressors, and have replaced the executioners with charitable brothers![25]

These sentiments were very much in line with a liberal re-envisioning of the Spanish nation in opposition to the myth of an Eternal Spain, derived from the Visigoths, the Catholic Kings, and Habsburg monarchs. This new vision identi-

---

23   "[D]ejando así la espiritual é inmortal á cargo de los Teologos y fijandome solo en los hechos que la esperiencia y la observacion dan de sí á los Medicos sobre eso se han ocupado." Ildefonso Martínez y Fernández, *Disertación leída al Ateneo Médico-Quirúrjico Matritense* (Madrid, 21 June 1840),BH AP 4, leg. 1, N° 7.

24   Martínez, *Médicos perseguidos*, 3. "No vamos ¡oh españoles! a recordar escenas sangrientas por gusto, vamos si á dar á conocer hechos poco conocidos, pero ciertos: atended y escarmentad, no en brazos de los mártires, sino en odio á los verdugos y tiranos del pensamiento. El pensamiento español perseguido por la Inquisición pudiera llenar muchos tomos, pero la institución de los reyes católicos, analizada médicamente, puede dar origen a grandes comentarios."

25   "¡Salud, oh grandes médicos perseguidos por la inquisicion: sí, salud, ilustres mártires; vosotros sufristeis los unos la encarcelacion, los otros el San Benito, algunos el destierro, otros la hoguera, pero vuestros comprofesores en la ciencia han hecho arrancar á vuestros tiranos infinitas víctimas, y les han dado en vez de verdugos caritativos hermanos!" Ibid., 94.

fied the true Spain with those persecuted for their beliefs, wrongly convicted, or forced into exile.[26] Of this liberal project, Jesús Torrecilla writes:

> Having rejected the official Spain, they came to identify with all those groups that had been victims of the authoritarianism and intolerance of their rulers. [...] Having been denied their Spanish identity by those who would monopolize it as if they were its only legitimate proprietors, they proposed, in turn, that the truly authentic Spain was constituted of precisely those groups that had been amputated from the common trunk for defending their beliefs: the persecuted, the exiles, those adjudicated in the name of a truth that was not their own. Moreover, in identifying with those groups, they projected onto them their own ideas, as if being victims of the same kind of intolerance created a sense of intellectual community among them.[27]

When it comes to early modern physicians as victims of the old regime, however, the 'intellectual community' that writers like Martínez perceived was, indeed, an imagined one. As Diego Gracia Guillén points out in an article entitled "Judaism, Medicine, and the Inquisitorial Mind in Sixteenth-Century Spain," while there is no doubt that physicians were persecuted by the Inquisition, they also collaborated with the Holy Office in pursuit of their own interests, and medical discourse played an important role in the widespread efforts to impose the social control that accompanied the rise of the early modern state. As Gracia Guillén puts it, "Medicine was a victim of the Inquisition, but it was also, and [...] to a larger extent, allied with the inquisitorial authorities in the task of corporally and morally disciplining sixteenth-century Spanish society."[28]

---

26 Henry Kamen has written on the role of exiles in Spanish history in *The Disinherited: Exile and the Making of Spanish Culture, 1492-1975* (New York, NY, 2007).

27 "El rechazo de la España oficial les lleva a identificarse con todos aquellos grupos que habían sido víctimas del autoritiarismo y la intolerancia de sus dirigentes. [...] Excluidos de la identidad española por los que pretendían monopolizar en exclusiva el espacio national, como si fueran sus unicos y legítimos propietarios, proponen a su vez que la España mas auténtica era precisamente la de aquellos grupos que habían sido amputados del tronco común por defender sus creencias, la de los perseguidos, exiliados y ajusticiados en nombre de una verdad que no era la suya. Ademas, al identificarse con esos grupos, proyectan sobre ellos sus ideas, como si el ser víctimas de una misma intolerancia estableciera entre ellos una comunidad de pensamiento." Jesús Torrecilla, *España al revés: Los mitos del pensamiento progresista (1790-1840)* (Madrid, 2016), 39-40.

28 Diego Gracia Guillén, "Judaism, Medicine, and the Inquisitorial Mind in Sixteenth-Century Spain," trans. Esther da Costa-Frankel, in *The Spanish Inquisition and the Inquisitorial*

How, then, did liberals such as Martínez reconstrue early modern medical discourse from a disciplinary force that buttressed church and monarchy into an emancipatory one that could support liberal political aspirations in the first half of the nineteenth century? In what follows, we will trace the course of this reimagining in some of the other works by Ildefonso Martínez y Fernández and his compatriots.

Another of Martínez's key examples of inquisitorial interference with the advancement of Spanish medicine was the censorship of Doctor Juan Huarte de San Juan's famous book, *Examen de ingenios* (*The Examination of Men's Wits,* Madrid, 1575). Huarte's work was a landmark in the history of psychology, representing the first attempt to account for psychological differences in physiological terms. The book was enormously popular and circulated throughout Europe in various translations. But Huarte's determinism and naturalism were hard to align with Catholic doctrines on free will and the immortality of the soul, and consequently his book was condemned by the Inquisition and had to be reissued in a revised edition in 1594.[29] In an attempt to right what he perceived to be a historical injustice, Martínez produced in 1846 a new Spanish edition of Huarte's work, restored for the first time to its original form, free from all inquisitorial expurgations.

Martínez's interest in Huarte de San Juan emerged from the same politico-scientific rifts within Spanish liberalism outlined above. The somatic determinism of Huarte's sixteenth-century treatise was very much in keeping with the phrenology of the nineteenth century and its localization of mental functions in the brain, and so Martínez's embrace of Huarte set him at odds with the vitalism of *moderado* physicians.[30] Indeed, Franz Joseph Gall drew on

---

Mind, 375-400, on 375. On the role of physicians in the Inquisition, see also José Pardo-Tomás and Alvar Martínez Vidal, "Victims and Experts: Medical Practitioners and the Spanish Inquisition," in John Woodward and Robert Jütte, eds., *Coping with Sickness: Medicine, Law and Human Rights. Historical Perspectives* (Sheffield, 2000), 11-27. For a comparative perspective, see Guido Ruggiero, "The Cooperation of Physicians and the State in the Control of Violence in Renaissance Venice," *Journal of the History of Medicine and Allied Sciences,* 33 (1978), 156-166.

29 On Huarte, see Malcolm K. Read, *Juan Huarte de San Juan* (Boston, MA, 1981). Ismael del Olmo argues that Huarte's naturalistic demonology actually served to square the circle with regard to the immortality of the soul. See "La posesión diabólica en el *Examen de ingenios para las sciencias* (1575) de Juan Huarte de San Juan: Una paradoja," *Tiempos modernos,* 8, no. 33 (2016), 70-101. See also, in this present volume, Guido Giglioni, "Between Galen and St Paul: How Juan Huarte de San Juan Responded to Inquisitorial Censorship."

30 This emphasis on the localization of mental functions presaged present-day cognitive

Huarte as an influence, a fact that Martínez emphasized in his introduction to his edition of the *Examen*.[31] In this same introduction, Martínez took aim at vitalist critics of Gall and Huarte, such as Laurent Cerise, the renowned French physician who had authored a widely read denunciation of phrenology.[32] Cerise's objection to phrenology stemmed from his vitalist conviction that the relationship between the physical and the moral could not be determined by brain functions alone. Instead, Cerise insisted that a 'vital energy' was distributed unevenly among men, and that this fact could account for the differences in human capacities that phrenology attributed to variations in brain anatomy.[33] Cerise singled out Huarte as a precursor to the materialism of the phrenologists, a materialism that conflicted with the spiritualist school of thought, which held that the soul was an autonomous immaterial entity, and that it could function independently from matter. Cerise went on to assert that Huarte's doctrines conflicted with Catholic orthodoxy, and that they represented "one of a thousand examples of the materialist consequences logically derived from a false science."[34] In response, Martínez suggested that Cerise was "too much of a spiritualist," and claimed that he had misconstrued Huarte's ideas, which, despite their naturalism, were, in fact, compatible with the teachings of the Church. Huarte did not deny the existence of an immaterial soul, but merely argued that it could only operate via physical organs. This was, as Martínez pointed out, not far removed from Cerise's own stance, and was compatible with the medical eclecticism of the day, which had sought to chart a middle way between materialism and spiritualism.[35]

---

scientists' focus on the modularity of mind. See Emilio García García, "Huarte de San Juan, un adelantado a la teoría modular de la mente," *Revista de historia de la psicología*, 24 (2003), 9-25.

31   Juan Huarte de San Juan, *Examen de ingenios para las ciencias,* ed. Ildefonso Martínez y Fernández (Madrid, 1846), xix.

32   Laurent Cerise, *Exposé et examen critique du système phrénologique: Considéré dans ses principes, dans sa méthode* (Brussels, 1837).

33   Williams, *The Physical and the Moral*, 221-222.

34   "Violà un example, entre mille, que nos pourrions citer, de la conséquence matérialiste tireé logiquement d'une science fausse [...]." Cerise, *Exposé*, 251.

35   "[P]ero si atendemos á que Cerise es demasiado espiritualista, á que él mismo dice que el hombre es una actividad espiritual que manda á una pasividad carnal sin ayuda de la que nada puede hacer, facilmente se deducirá que estuvo algun tanto inconsecuente al atacar á Huarte." Huarte, *Examen*, xxxi. On the influence of eclecticism in France, see Williams, *The Physical and the Moral*, 140-151; and John I. Brooks, *The Eclectic Legacy: Academic Philosophy and the Human Sciences in Nineteenth-Century France* (Newark, NJ, 1998). The

While Huarte the scientist might elicit contention within the wider milieu of Spanish liberalism, Huarte the medical martyr was a unifying figure. For Martínez, he was a valuable addition to his catalogue of physicians who had suffered at the hands of the Inquisition; he referred to him as "a martyr for the freedom of philosophy," which was a sentiment upon which liberals of all stripes could agree.[36] An example of this sentiment was captured in verse by Martínez's friend and fellow liberal, Ricardo López Arcilla. In the poem, Arcilla extolled the virtues of the *Examen* and denounced the Inquisition's treatment of Huarte. He described the "sublime *Examen*" as an "immortal book that the nations of the world proudly translate into their own languages and never cease to admire," and lauded Huarte as the recipient of "a gigantic flame" that the Lord had ignited in his "magnificent and splendid mind."[37] The Spanish Inquisition, in contrast, he characterized as

> That horrendous tribunal
> Of evils and injustices
> Presiding with malice
> In all its acts;
> Detested by all
> For its iniquitous covenants,
> The *Examen de Ingenios*
> Was sullied by its black hand.
> And tearing out pages of sublime orations
> That described the passions
> Of the divine Redeemer,
> It extended its dark shadows
> Over the earthly sojourn
> Augmenting the ignorance
> That it was designed to protect.[38]

French physician Victor Cousin was one representative of this school who was highly influential in Spain. See Rey González, "Juan Bautista Peset y Vidal," 89.

36   Huarte, *Examen*, xxxii.

37   "Es un rayo tan solo desprendido de la gigante llama que el soplo del Señor hubo encendido en tu mente magnífica y grandiosa que el genio del hombre poderosa El Examen sublime ha producido. Ese libro inmortal que las naciones con orgullo traducen en su idioma […]." Ricardo López Arcilla, "A Huarte: Composición dedicada al doctor D. Ildefonso Martínez," BH AP 4, leg. 2, N⁰ 29.

38   "Ese tribunal horrendo / De maldades é injusticias / A quien siempre la malicia / En sus actos presidió; / A quien todos detestamos / Por sus inicuos convenios, / En el *Examen de Yngenios* / Su negra mano estampó. / Y rasgando algunas hojas / De sublimes oraciones /

Arcilla concluded his poem with a paean to Huarte as a harbinger of liberal values, and with a tribute to Martínez for his editorial acumen, praising his edition of the *Examen* as a tribute to "holy liberty," and urging Martínez to continue his struggle to ensure that "the light of reason is not clouded by the forces of slander and error."[39]

Martínez himself wrote in praise of Huarte in an article that appeared in the *Círculo Científico y Literario*, a prominent journal of the medical press.[40] There he portrayed Huarte as the quintessential liberal reformer, whose critiques of the existing social order brought him into conflict with the vested interests of his day. Because he wrote on "the qualities that a king should have, not to mention what characteristics are required of judges, priests, physicians, and all the social classes," and because he dedicated himself to "attacking entrenched prejudices, censuring abuses, and exploring a path no one had tread before him," Huarte was, in Martínez's estimation, unfairly targeted by those whose privileges he threatened. Martínez lamented that Huarte wrote during "an epoch in which inquisitorial power was in full force," and speculated that if he had lived in more favorable times, his doctrines would not have raised an eyebrow.[41]

But while the Inquisition's censorship of Huarte gained him entry into Martínez's pantheon of liberal heroes, in reality Huarte's doctrines did not fit easily with liberal notions of religious toleration and equality before the law. As Gracia Guillén illustrates, Huarte insisted on the primacy of temperament – that is to say, the balance of Galenic humors – in the determination of all human abilities and the capacity to learn, and while this extreme biological determinism may have caused him trouble with the Inquisition, it was ultimately mobilized in support of the hierarchical social structure of the old regime and exerted a profound influence on the moral discourse of early modern Spain.

Que pintaban las pasiones / Del divino Redentor, / Estendió sus negras sombras / Por la terrenal estancia / Aumentando la ignorancia / De la que era protector." Ibid.

39   "Que la luz de la razón no la empañan las tinieblas de la injuria y del error." Ibid.

40   Ildefonso Martínez y Fernández, "Juan Huarte," *Círculo Científico y Literario*, 4 (1854), 84-90.

41   "En tan desgraciada época y cuando el poder inquisitorial estaba mas en fuerza, es cuando Huarte se lanza á escribir un *Exámen de Ingénios* y á dedicar un articulo exclusivamente para representar las cualidades de que debiera estar dotado un Rey, sin dejar de manifestar las muchas condiciones que exigian los jurisperitos, los sacerdotes, los medicos y todas las clases sociales, atacando preocupaciones arraigadas, tachando abusos y penetrando una senda aun desconocida hasta él, teniendo que compaginar por el esfuerzo de su ingenio muchas cosas que si hubiera escrito en época mas bonancible no se hubiera curado ni aun de justificarlas." Ibid., 89.

Huarte's influence manifested itself in two important and interconnected ways. The first of these was as a support for the anti-Semitism that permeated early modern Spain. The idea, so prevalent in Huarte, that moral qualities were rooted in biology, and thus heritable, became a standard trope in debates about the status of the Jews and figured prominently in the construction of a racial caste system. Archbishop Juan Martínez Siliceo, a figure instrumental in the promulgation of the purity of blood statutes, compared Spain to a stable in which inferior breeds of horses must be culled from the herd.[42] Such was the power of Jewish blood that, by the second half of the sixteenth century, inquisitors were convinced that Judaizing could be instigated by the mere fact of having a Jewish wet nurse.[43]

A second trend to which Huarte contributed was the development of a "medical political" literature in early modern Spain that emphasized "with an energy not seen since the times of Greece and Rome, [...] 'constitutional factors' in the determination of human actions."[44] According to Gracia Guillén, during the sixteenth century, "while the Inquisition was becoming 'medicalized,' medicine in its turn, was becoming aware of its enormous political potential and its power as a disciplinarian of human conduct."[45] This new awareness inspired a long list of treatises purporting to derive political insight from the structure of the human body and the practice of medicine. A host of such works proliferated during the sixteenth century, such as Enrique Jorge Enríquez's *Retrato del perfecto médico* (*Portrait of the Perfect Physician,* Salamanca, 1595), Jerónimo Merola's *República original sacada del cuerpo humano* (*Original Republic Derived from the Human Body*, Barcelona, 1587), and Oliva Sabuco de Nantes' *Nueva filosofía de la naturaleza del hombre* (*New Philosophy of Human Nature*, Madrid, 1588), which Martínez released in a new edition in 1847. The seventeenth century saw the publication of similar works, including Rodrigo de Castro's *Medicus politicus* (*The Political Physician*, Hamburg, 1614) and Cosme Gil Negrete's *Conclusiones medico politicae* (*Medico-Political Conclusions*, Madrid, 1654). Many of these books refer to Huarte by name, and all of them follow the idea that moral and social behaviors are determined by physiological processes, and that the physician could therefore intervene in order to control these behaviors, and in doing so govern the microcosm of the human body – just as the prince governed the mesocosm of the republic, and God the macrocosm of the world.[46]

---

42   Gracia Guillén, "Judaism, Medicine," 382.
43   Ibid., 384.
44   Ibid., 379.
45   Ibid., 384-385.
46   Ibid., 389.

Oliva Sabuco de Nantes uses precisely this sort of language in her *Nueva filosofía*, referring to the human body as 'the small world' and using it as a touchstone for part three of the work, entitled *"Coloquio de las cosas que mejoran este mundo y sus repúblicas"* (Colloquium on the Things That Improve This World and Its Republics).[47] The physician, according to Sabuco, is the "minister of the great secrets that God – and His secondary cause, nature – have created," and he must exercise his profession "with equity and justice," thereby "eschewing all that is misguided and injurious and substituting what is correct and useful for his patients and for the republic."[48] One important way the physician can serve the republic is through an understanding of heredity. In a chapter on marriage, Sabuco decries the common tendency to base marriages on economic factors and to forget that "the principle of perfecting human nature, as we see every day, is that the faults of the parents are seen in the children."[49] In this emphasis on the hereditary nature of moral qualities, Sabuco's medico-political doctrines approximate Huarte's, as Martínez points out in a footnote in his edition of the *Nueva filosofía*.[50] Sabuco closes the chapter with a passage of which Huarte would have approved: "When we desire a good horse, we go in search of a fine stud. Should we not likewise examine the man who would become a father and grandfather, so that he has good children and descendants, able men, and not beasts?"[51]

The doctrine that the heritability of physiological traits determined moral and spiritual qualities is also evident in Enrique Jorge Enríquez's *Retrato del*

---

47   Oliva Sabuco de Nantes Barrera, *Nueva filosofía de la naturaleza del hombre, no conocida ni alcanzada de los grandes filósofos antiquos, la cual mejora la vida y la salud humana,* ed. Ildefonso Martínez y Fernández (Madrid, 1847), 450. The authorship of the *Nueva filosofía* was transferred to Oliva's father, Miguel, after documents were discovered in 1903 purporting to show that Miguel Sabuco had actually written the work. Historians, however, continue to debate the issue. See, for example, María C. Vintró and Mary Ellen Waithe, *¿Fue Oliva o fue Miguel?: Reconsiderando el caso Sabuco* (México, D.F., 2000).

48   "[P]ues el médico es el ministro de las grandezas y secretos que Dios y su causa segunda la naturaleza criaron." "Y asi suplico á los sábios y cristianos médicos juzguen este negocio con equidad y justicia, pues les hacemos bien, y no mal, quitando lo errado y nocivo, y dándoles lo acertado y útil para ellos y para las repúblicas." Sabuco, *Nueva filosofía,* 480-481.

49   "Pues no es menor yerro el que el vulgo hace cada dia en los casamientos, no mirando mas de la hacienda y riqueza, olvidando lo principal que es la perfeccion de naturaleza en la persona, como se ve cada dia, y es cosa notoria ver las faltas de los padres en los hijos." Ibid., 470.

50   Ibid., 473, n.

51   "Buscas y examinas un caballo para padre por tener buenos caballos, y ¿no examinarás al hombre que ha de ser padre de tus nietos y descendientes, para tener buenos nietos y decendientes, hombres habiles y no bestias?" Ibid., 475.

perfecto médico, a work that draws on Huarte explicitly. In keeping with his immersion in the tradition of Greek medicine epitomized by Galen and Hippocrates, Enríquez holds that the moral qualities of a physician are determined by his physical appearance: "The physician who has a handsome face cannot but be capable and skilled and have other qualities that are necessary for the perfect physician, since it is a philosophical rule that the customs of the soul follow the temper and complexion of the body, as Galen has shown in his book."[52]

As with the physician, so too with the king. Enríquez warns against monarchs with badly organized humors, as their hearts will tend towards irascibility, which when joined with great power is a dangerous thing.[53] The familiar equation of physician and king is a recurrent theme with Enríquez; both enjoy "great power" and have "subjects." The physician is king of the *pequeño mundo* of the body just as the monarch is the ruler of the republic.[54] Medicine as a political science, then, has the goal of examining the relationship between the corporeal order of the body and the political order of the republic. This goal can be clearly seen in Cosmo Gil Negrete's *Conclusiones medico politicae.* In it he sets out to establish "the brotherhood between politics and medicine;" he points out that "some kings of Egypt chose the study of medicine, and in particular the study of anatomy," and states his conviction that "they included in this course of study the politics of governing, because in the parts of the human body we see the parts of a republic."[55] Not surprisingly, as the treatise was written in honor of King Philip IV, the prince corresponds to the heart of the body politic, while the tongue corresponds to the royal councilors, the hands are the executive ministers, the feet are the peasants, and so on and so forth, all bound together in hierarchical fashion, as befits an absolute monarchy.

---

52   "Y mas que el Medico que fuere de rostro hermoso, no podra dexar de tener buena habilidad, è ingenio, y otras partes, que son necessarias para vno ser perfecto Medico, que regla es de philosophia que las costumbres del alma siguen el temple y complexion de cuerpo, como Galeno lo muestra en vn libro." Enrique Jorge Enríquez, *Retrato del perfecto médico* (Salamanca, 1595), 147; Quoted by Gracia Guillén, "Judaism, Medicine," 389-390.

53   Enríquez, *Retrato,* 50; Gracia Guillén, "Judaism, Medicine," 393.

54   "[E]stavan obligados a hazer los Reyes y principes passados para auer de gouernar el mundo: y porque no lo haran los Medicos para regir el cuerpo del hombre que se llama mundo pequeño." Enríquez, *Retrato,* 31; Gracia Guillén, "Judaism, Medicine," 393.

55   "Conclvsion IIII. Hermandad de la politica, y la medicina. Algunos Reyes de Egipto, de la medicina, eligieron por estudio, la parte que toca a la anatomia; y me persuado, que no dexaron en este estudio el politico de gouernar, porque en las partes del cuerpo humano, se ven las de vna republica." Doctor Cosme Gil Negrete, "Conclusiones medico politicae Philippo IIII" (Madrid, 1654), 7-8.

As Gracia Guillén has demonstrated, this genre of medico-political literature was widespread in early modern Spain; but it endured well into the nineteenth century. In 1855, for example, Ildefonso Martínez y Fernández followed
in the footsteps of Enrique Jorge Enríquez with a work entitled, *Espejo del verdadero médico* (*Mirror of the True Physician*). Martínez's work appropriates the
structure of its early modern predecessor, but with some crucial differences.
Enríquez, as we have seen, insisted on a strict parallelism between physical
and moral qualities, an insistence that Gracia Guillén links to racism and anti-
Semitism:

> This moral biologism naturally led to racism, that is, to the differentiation
> between noble and ignoble families, good and bad families, only by their
> blood or name. In reality this doctrine, which has in Huarte its major
> exponent, served to differentiate families by their blood. This suited the
> monarchy and nobility perfectly, and they gladly took advantage of it.
> The theme of blood served not only to isolate the Jews and Moriscos but
> to sanctify the nobles and kings as 'bluebloods.'[56]

Given the decidedly illiberal slant of certain aspects of the medico-political
literature, what was a good liberal to do? Martínez's solution seems to have
been to tweak a number of these medico-political tropes. For example, where
Enríquez argues that the perfect physician must be an attractive physical specimen, Martínez demurs. He writes that "when it comes to the physical qualities
of the physician, we do not wish to say that he must be a model of physical
perfection; we will not delineate an Adonis, but we will rather speak of the
physical requirements that are indispensible for ease and comfort in exercising
his profession." He goes on to assure his readers that a good physician can be
"beautiful or ugly, tall or short, fat or skinny, straight-spined or humpbacked,
hairy or bald."[57]

   In another instance of selective appropriation, Martínez adopts a format
typical of the medico-political literature, but he eschews the latent anti-Semitism of the genre, choosing to write the *Espejo* under a Jewish pseudonym:
Rabbi Isaac Maimon Firdusi. The Rabbi, tellingly, shares the same initials as

---

56   Gracia Guillén, "Judaism, Medicine," 391.

57   "Al examinar las cualidades físicas del médico, no queremos decir que sea un portento de
      perfeccion física; no vamos a delinear un Adonis, sino que hablamos de las condiciones
      físicas indispensables, necesarias para el fácil, cómodo y beneficioso ejercicio de la profe-
      sion." Rabbi Isaac Maimon Firdusi [Ildefonso Martínez y Fernández], *Espejo del verdadero
      médico* (Madrid, 1855), 14.

Martínez, and some of the same political tendencies as well. He writes that "although I am a rabbi, I am tolerant – so much so that the second book of this work is a direct translation of a Catholic author, whose views on the role of religion in the life of a physician I could not bring myself to alter."[58] The rabbi goes on to decry the anti-Semitic stereotypes often aimed at Jewish physicians and then to declare a deep affiliation with Spain: "Jew that I am, when I speak of Spanish authors I refer to them as 'ours' because I am directly descended from Maimones de Lara of Spain, and although, as a Jew, I wander without a homeland, I will always take Spain as my own."[59] The sentiments of Martínez's alter ego capture perfectly the aforementioned tendency of Spanish liberals to dispute the master narrative of a centralized, racially pure Spain, and to substitute in its stead an emphasis on medieval *convivencia* and regional autonomy. Martínez's choice of a Jewish pseudonym underscores his identification with the persecuted and the exiled – all those whom he saw as victims of intolerance, those who had become martyrs for their beliefs.

Even when Martínez deals with Catholicism itself, he takes pains to display a tolerant and ecumenical stance. While conceding that a physician should be a faithful and orthodox Catholic, he adds in the same breath that

> the religion of the physician is *humanity*, the universal religion that takes man as the object of its study and meditations. He must be nothing less than tolerant toward all, and by the same token, whatever religion a physician may profess, he should fulfill his duty, if he indeed knows what it means to be religious – that is to say, *human*, and charitable in every sense of the word; *in omnibus charitas*, to quote St. Augustine.[60]

Just as the 'mirror of the physician' endured into the nineteenth century as a literary genre, so too did the 'body politic' as metaphor, but again, with some significant adaptations. Another publication in the vibrant medical press of

---

58   "Aunque rabino soy tolerante, y tanto, que habiendo traducido integro el segundo libro de esta obra de un autor católico, no quise molestarme en rehacerle respecto á lo que dice de la religion del médico." Ibid., v.

59   "Judio como soy, hablando de los autores españoles, les llamo nuestros, porque desciendo por linea recta de los Maimones de Lara de España; y aunque, como judio, *errante y sin patria*, llevo y tengo siempre á España por la mia." Ibid., vi.

60   "[L]a religion del médico es la *humanidad*: religion universal que, basada en el hombre, objeto de su estudio y de sus meditaciones, no puede menos de ser *tolerante* con todas, y por lo mismo, sea cualquiera la que profese el médico, llegará á, cumplir con su deber si sabe ser religioso, esto es, *humano*, caritativo en toda la estension de la palabra; *in omnibus charitas*, que dijo San Agustin." Ibid., 93.

the nineteenth century was *El Porvenir Médico* (*The Medical Future*), and Martínez was a frequent contributor. He was joined in his contributions by a number of like-minded colleagues, and together they offered up a wide-ranging critique of the status quo, both medical and political. One such colleague, by the name of Juan Amich, wrote in the edition of September 25th, 1854 a piece entitled *"La medicina y la política"* ("Medicine and Politics").[61] In it, Amich translates the traditional, hierarchical body politic metaphor, used by authors such as Negrete, into one more suitable for a constitutional government. Here the human body is a 'confederation' subject to the legislation of natural law. Man is not a cause, according to Amich, but rather an effect of this natural law, which can be seen as a legislative power outside ourselves, imbuing us with our functions and capacities, all of which are constrained by a strict separation of powers – our limbs cannot usurp the power of our vision any more than the digestive system can take the place of the intellect. Continuing, Amich declares that

> the executive power [is] situated in the superior part of our being, the intelligence, with the nervous system putting it in relation to the exterior. The administrative order is divided between two great functionaries: the digestive tract with its lymphatic vessels that carry the liquids destined for the nutrition of the body, and the central circulatory system. It is this center that receives the sanction of the legislative power and is responsible for discharging it via the arteries, and thereby assimilating it throughout the entire economy. What we have here, then, are limitations on executive power, and the administration subject to the power of the legislature.[62]

So, instead of the traditional use of the metaphor to legitimate absolutism, Amich uses it to advocate a cooperative, harmonious body politic, governed according to checks and balances.

---

61 *El Porvenir Médico: Periódico oficial de las Academias Quirúgicas Matritense y Cesaragus-tana*, no. 107 (Madrid, Sept. 25, 1854), 211-212.

62 "El ejecutivo colocado en su parte superior, tal es la intelegencia, con los cordones nervi-osos que la ponen en relacion consigo mismo y con el esterior. El órden administrativo que lo constituyen dos grandes funcionarios, el aparato digetivo con sus vasos linfáticos y venosos que llevan los liquidos destinados á la nutricion, el centro del aparato circulato-rio; y este centro que recibe la sancion del poder legislativo encarandose luego de que por medio de los conductos arteriales, se efectue la asimilacion en toda nuestra economia, es decir, el poder ejecutivo limitado y la administracion, parte del legislativo." Ibid., 212.

Continuing along these lines, Amich emphasizes the need for popular sovereignty, meaning "a number of individuals elected by the people and for the people, with the power to legislate, organize the administration, and name public functionaries, including the executive power." It is only through popular oversight of the executive power that the "the harmony, health, and life of the people" can be assured, and a lack of such oversight will inevitably lead to the "sickness and death of the nation."[63] Constant vigilance must be exercised in order to avoid the depredations of excessive executive power, according to Amich:

> We must declaw the lion so that we will no longer be afraid. The claws of executive power consist in the ability to avail itself of the public goods of the country in an almost absolute fashion, thus giving rise to a rabid thirst for riches that will bring about the misery of the people, and once these riches are secured, they will be used to generously reward those in the employ of the executive, so that they become faithful servants of their master.[64]

The only bulwark against this state of affairs in Amich's view is the appointment of autonomous public functionaries who cannot be dismissed for partisan reasons. And what if, despite these safeguards, a public functionary becomes a creature of the executive power? In a final corporeal metaphor, Amich warns that such a creature must immediately be excised from the body politic before his "sickness threatens his fellow functionaries."[65]

The preceding foray into the uses of medical discourse in the political realm has shown that medico-political literature was not unique to the early modern era and has examined some of the ways in which interactions between medicine and the Inquisition fueled the nineteenth-century political imagination

---

63   "Consideremos á el pueblo soberano: representada su soberania por un número de individuos elegidos del pueblo y por el pueblo con la facultad de legislar, ordenar la administracion y nombrar los funcionarios públicos incluso el poder ejecutivo." "[S]olo asi comprendemos la armonia, la salud y la vida de los pueblos, de lo contrario la inmoralidad y en consecuencia la enfermedad y la muerte del pais." Ibid.

64   "Quitemos las garras al leeon y le perderemos el temor. Las garras del poder ejecutivo consisten en esa facultad que se le concede de disponer casi de un modo absoluto de los bienes de la patria y de sus administrativos, resultando de ahí que su insaciable hidrópica sed de oro puede dar por resultado la miseria de todo el pueblo, y con el mismo oro retribuir con prodigalidad á sus empleados, convirtiendoles en fieles servidores de su señor [...]." Ibid.

65   "[A]pliquemos pues tambien el pronto remedio antes de que conmine el mal á los demas funcionarios." Ibid.

in Spain. The prevalence of physicians as both medical practitioners and literary figures within Spanish liberalism invites further analysis of the role of medicine – both as a science and as a metaphor – in the building of nations and the construction of a nationalist ideology, and may thus make some contribution toward filling the lacuna in the research on nationalism identified by Warwick and Pols, as well as opening up avenues for further comparative study.[66]

As a science, medicine functioned as a vehicle for criticizing the old regime, not only for its alleged mistreatment of physicians, but also for its failure to modernize. In addition to the topics that have been discussed thus far, Martínez put forth his ideas for reforming the Spanish state in a number of tracts that advocated new roles for the the medical profession, presenting the physician as a ubiquitous technocrat who "like Proteus, is multiplied into a thousand forms."[67] According to Martínez, physicians should oversee

> charitable institutions, the creation of hospitals, orphanages, maternity wards, insane asylums, the penitentiary system, correctional institutions, jails, penitentiaries, poor houses (with regard to the number of inhabitants and what kinds of food and drink are provided), the building of military barracks, naval stations and commercial ports, the construction of theaters and all recreational establishments, houses of prostitution, churches and cemeteries, physical and moral education for the youth of both sexes, and hygiene regimens for schools.[68]

And as if that portfolio were not enough, Martínez's ideal physician should also be prepared to "give reports, consultations, opinions, advice, and other documentation, either orally or in writing, to municipal councils and even the government," with the ultimate goal being to "serve the state loyally as a good man and virtuous citizen."[69]

---

66 See above, note 5.

67 "[E]s un Proteo, se multiplica bajo mil formas." Martínez, *Espejo del perfecto médico,* 154.

68 "[C]asas de beneficencia, creation de hospitales, hospicios, casas de maternidad, casas de locos, sistema penitenciario, casas de correccion, cárceles, presidios, causas [sic] del pauperismo y proporcion de subsistencias con el número de habitantes, clase de alimentos y bebidas considerados en general, creation de cuarteles y usos militares, apostaderos de marina y viages marítimos, construccion de teatros y todo género de establecimientos placenteros, casas de prostitution, iglesias y cementerios, educacion física y moral de la juventud de ambos sexos, y como su consecuencia los colegios y su regimen higiénico." Ibid.

69 "[D]ar informes, consultas, dictámenes, consejos y otros documentos por escrito ó de palabra á las corporacions municipales, provinciales y aun al gobierno [...]." "[S]ervir al Estado con la lealtad de un hombre de bien y de un virtuoso ciudadano." Ibid., 160.

When it comes to medicine as metaphor, this essay has traced the body politic metaphor into the nineteenth century, and in so doing invites further comparative investigation into its persistence in European political thought. In England, for example, Peter Elmer has shown that, contrary to the traditional scholarly consensus, the organicist notion of the state endured well beyond the English Civil War of the 1640s, and that far from representing an inherently conservative politics, "parallels drawn between human and political bodies might as easily articulate criticism of the status quo as [...] slavish acceptance of the traditional political order."[70] This certainly accords with what we have seen in nineteenth-century Spain, where such a critical articulation of the body politic metaphor can be found in liberal political discourse.

An additional direction for further study has to do with the nature of metaphor itself. When we speak of metaphor, it is tempting to conceive of it as superfluous to the real work of thought, a poetical oversimplification of more abstract concepts. But as George Lakoff and Mark Johnson have argued, metaphors are central to human cognition and are rooted in embodied experience rather than in some Platonic realm of pure form.[71] From this perspective, the metaphor of the body politic is not a quaint rhetorical flourish or a mere ornamentation of legitimate political theory; it must be seen, rather, as integral to the way humans conceptualize social relationships. With the aid of conceptual metaphor theory it should be possible to link culture and cognition by tracing how the body as a source domain has changed over time in the context of our cultural history and thereby go beyond a mere cataloguing of textual references.[72]

Recognizing the power and ubiquity of metaphor is not meant to elide the reality it refers to. Having examined the role of medical metaphors in the

---

70   Peter Elmer, *Medicine and Politics in Early Modern Britain* (Oxford, forthcoming). See ch. 2, "The Premature Death of a Renaissance Commonplace: The Body Politic in Puritan England, 1640-1660."

71   See George Lakoff and Mark Johnson, *Metaphors We Live By*, 2nd ed. (Chicago, IL, 2003), and eidem, *Philosophy in the Flesh: The Embodied Mind and Its Challenge to Western Thought* (New York, NY, 1999).

72   Andreas Musolff sketches a possible approach in, "Political Metaphor and Bodies Politic," in Urszula Okulska and Piotr Cap, eds., *Discourse Approaches to Politics, Society and Culture* (Amsterdam, 2010), 37. "The project of writing a history of the body politic metaphor that goes beyond the mere chronological listing of texts in which it appears can thus be written on the basis of a cooperation between cognitive semantics, conceptual history and critical discourse analysis. Cognitive analysis can establish, through investigation of conceptual mappings, the semantic elements that provide the source inputs for the metaphor."

political discourse of Spanish liberalism, we must not lose sight of the very real bodies and governing institutions that ultimately gave rise to a different, and more deadly, form of medical politics. The political reforms envisioned by Spanish liberals were not thwarted merely by competing ideologies with better metaphors, but rather by social chaos due to food shortages caused by poor harvests and ill-considered government policies. These factors, in turn, led to unrest in the countryside and contributed to the scourge of cholera that wracked the Iberian peninsula intermittently throughout the nineteenth century.[73] In 1854, for example, the radical faction of the liberal coalition seized power in a revolutionary uprising and was determined to finally redress the injustices facing *campesinos* in rural Spain. Their efforts were undermined, however, by an outbreak of cholera that brought to ruin not only hopes of progressive liberal governance in Spain, but also Ildefonso Martínez y Fernández himself.[74]

The theme of martyrdom runs throughout Martínez's career. Returning to where we began, with his historical sketch on the Spanish Inquisition, we see Martínez celebrating physicians who were persecuted not only for their defense of scientific ideals, but also for their commitment to free inquiry. Summarizing his views toward the end of his treatise, Martínez writes

> This has been the history of the physicians who were persecuted by the Spanish Inquisition – worthy and illustrious men who were victimized because of their science [...]. And after all of this, and the great torments they inflicted, the inquisitors failed to see that instead of killing the idea, instead of destroying the mind that created it, the idea passed from the mind of one man into the mind of humanity. [...] Oh, what holy foolishness it is, this attempt to suppress moral concepts through physical torture! One's hair stands on end when thinking of the martyrs that the inquisitions have made in the name of authority and against the freedom of inquiry.[75]

---

73   Charles J. Esdaile, *Spain in the Liberal Age: From Constitution to Civil War, 1808-1939* (Oxford, 2000), 69.

74   Ibid., 106.

75   "Esta es la historia de los médicos que han sido perseguidos por la Inquisición Española, víctimas ilustres y dignas, porque lo fueron de su ciencia [...]. Y despues de todo esto y de los grandes tormentos no han visto los inquisidores que en vez de matar la idea, que en vez de concluir con el cerebro que la habia creado, la idea pasó del cerebro de un hombre al cerebro de la humanidad. ¡Oh santa simplicidad! que bien puede llamarse así querer ahogar las ideas morales por los tormentos físicos. Los cabellos se erizan al ver la multitud

Martínez clearly saw himself as an heir to the idealism of these persecuted physicians who were willing to sacrifice themselves in the service of their professional calling. He sought to reform both an antiquated system of public health and the political system of the old regime, but like many other reformers, Martínez ended up disillusioned by the failure of the liberal project and finally became a victim of his own idealism. In his *Espejo del verdadero médico*, Martínez reprised the theme of martyrdom, exhorting his fellow physicians to emulate their historical counterparts and to "live as martyrs in order to die virtuously," and in a chapter on plagues and epidemics he wrote that "the primary duty of the physician during epidemics and contagions is to aid the sick valorously, to never abandon the victims no matter how numerous they may be, and no matter how dangerous and deadly are the symptoms they present."[76] True to his convictions, in 1855 Martínez traveled to his native Asturias to treat victims of the cholera epidemic. Shortly after his arrival, he contracted the disease himself and died in Oviedo at the age of 34.

---

de mártires que las inquisiciones han hecho a nombre de la autoridad contra el libre exámen." Martínez, *Médicos perseguidos*, 84-85.

76   "[Á] vivir mártires para morir virtuosos[…]." Martínez, *Espejo*, 13. "El primero de todos los deberes del médico en las epidemias y contagios, es la asistencia á los enfermos, es el valor que no abandona á las víctimas por numerosas que sean, ni por peligrosos y mortíferos que se presenten los síntomas." Ibid., 131.

"Speaking with the Fire": The Inquisition Confronts Mesoamerican Divination to Treat Child Illness in Sixteenth-Century Guatemala

Martha Few
Pennsylvania State University
mzf52@psu.edu

Abstract

Indigenous midwives and female healers who treated infants and children in late-six-teenth-century Guatemala were medico-religious specialists who mediated the natural and supernatural realms to treat child illness. Their socially critical roles are examined through the lens of an Inquisition investigation in the tributary Maya town of Samayaq in colonial Central America into indigenous and mixed race women's use of divination as a strategy to treat child illness, and in particular *mollera caída,* or fallen fontanel.

Keywords

female healers – divination – child illness – fallen fontanel – Inquisition – Maya Indians – Guatemala – Latin America

Sometime during 1595 in the small tributary Maya town of Samayaq, which was located west of Santiago de Guatemala, the capital of colonial Central America, an infant boy named Alonso became gravely ill from *mollera caída* (fallen fontanel), which referred to damage caused to the soft part of the skull

* Department of History, 108 Weaver Building, University Park, PA 16802, USA. The author would like to thank Maria Pia Donato and the two anonymous reviewers, whose comments and suggestions have significantly strengthened this essay.

of a fetus or infant between the frontal and parietal bones.[1] To those who cared for Alonso, he seemed on the verge of death. His mother, Doña María Velásquez, had hired the well-known *mulata* curers Isabel de Abrego and her adult daughter María de Abrego to treat the infant.[2] As Alonso's symptoms worsened, Velásquez also hired a local wet nurse named Catalina Sánchez to breastfeed him.[3] Nothing, however, seemed to improve the boy's condition.

Isabel de Abrego told Velásquez that it was time to send for two indigenous female healers she knew, who specialized in treating infants, to come to the house, describing them as "two old Indian women, named in their maternal languages Atichivalan and Atixiguite."[4] Atichivalan (whom we later learn, after her arrest and imprisonment, was also called Isabel Chivalan) treated the boy first. She used a combination of ritual divination, prayers and the physical manipulation of the skull, inside of the mouth, and of the feet and toes – actions that together were designed to "raise the boy's fontanel."[5] Atixiguite (whose Hispanicized name was recorded as Isabel Roche Giguir) came to the house a few days later and performed a similar combination of divinatory acts and pressure on various body parts to treat Alonso. One of the healers ritually prophesized that the boy would die from his illness, the other's divination demonstrated that he would live. Later testimony showed that he eventually

---

1   I am grateful to Christopher Lutz for bringing this case to my attention, and to Brad Bouley for inviting me to contribute to this volume. Archivo General de la Nación (Mexico City, Mexico), Ramo de Inquisición (hereafter AGN, Inq.), vol. 209, exp. 2, ff. 1r-33r. This disease can also be referred to as *caída de la mollera*. In the sixteenth century Samayaq was located in the provincia de Zapotitlán y Suchitepéquez in the *Audiencia* of Guatemala, a geographic area that stretched from what is today Chiapas (in Mexico) through much of modern-day Central America. I have updated the spelling for "fontanel," though I do retain the spelling "fontanelle" in titles and in quotes from secondary sources where appropriate.

2   In this essay I follow the racial-ethnic designations used by notaries to describe those who appear in Inquisition cases, such as "Indian" (*yndio/a*); "Spaniard" (*español/a*); "Black" (*negro/a*). In colonial Central America, "*mestizo/a*" was used to refer to a person of mixed Spanish and indigenous parentage, and "*mulato/a*" to a person of mixed Spanish, indigenous, and/or African parentage. For more on racial/ethnic designations used in colonial Guatemala, see W. George Lovell and Christopher H. Lutz, eds., *Demography and Empire: A Guide to the Population History of Spanish Central America, 1500-1821* (Boulder, CO, 1995). In the main text I have updated spellings of names and added accents. I retain the original orthography in quotes from the primary sources.

3   Catalina Sánchez was listed a resident of Samayaq, married to Juan de León Cardona. The notary did not record her age or ethnicity in the Inquisition documents.

4   "[D]os yndias viejas llamadas en la lengua materna Atichivalan y Atixiguite," AGN, Inq. vol. 209, exp. 2, ff. 1r-33r: f. 3r. All translations are my own unless otherwise noted in the text.

5   "[A]lzaron la mollera del niño," AGN, Inq. vol. 209, exp. 2, f. 29r.

recovered his health.[6] María de Abrega, in her testimony under questioning about sorcery, neatly summed up Atichivalan and Atiguite's acts as simple healing and nothing more, that the fontanel had fallen and the healers had elevated it.[7]

Guatemala's Inquisition became formally involved after an unnamed person, clearly familiar with the details of the infant Alonso's illness and treatment, travelled to Santiago de Guatemala and informed Don Francisco González, the bishopric's judge provisor in charge of the Inquisition there, of the women's use of divination for healing. González named Father Alonso Gutiérrez, a priest and curate from a town near Samayaq, San Antonio Suchitepéquez, to head the investigation, hire a notary and indigenous language translators, and purchase paper and other supplies.[8] He authorized Gutiérrez to investigate all the mixed race and indigenous women in the area who used "divinations and sorceries and superstitions and spell casting" as central parts of their ritual healing practices.[9] A total of seven female healers from Samayaq and the surrounding small towns, representing various ritual-medical specialties, were arrested and imprisoned as a result of the Inquisition's investigations. They included the *mulata* mother and daughter Isabel de Abrego and María de Abrego and five indigenous women: Isabel Chivalan (alias Atichivalan), Isabel Roche Giguir (alias Atixiguite), Catalina Hune, Isabel Juaniha and Catalina Chirincoa.

Information on Mesoamerican religious and divinatory practices related to illness and medicine tends to enter the archival records only when civil, criminal, and Inquisition officials elected to police them. In the sixteenth century, Guatemala's Inquisition attempted to shape and contest Mesoamerican medical cultures by discounting them as ineffective, or by characterizing the activities of indigenous and mixed race healers in terms of practices of the occult.[10] This perspective has carried over into histories of science and medicine in colonial Latin America and the Spanish Empire where, until recently, indigenous medical cultures have largely been ignored, or when noted, represented as

---

6   Ibid., f. 4r.

7   Ibid., f. 21v.

8   Ibid., 2, f. 33r-v.

9   "[Q]ue usan de adivinas y sortilegas y de supersticiones y hechizerias," ibid., f. 1r.

10   For the history of the early Inquisition see, for example, Solange Alberro, *Inquisición y sociedad en México, 1571-1700* (Mexico, 1988); Jorge Traslosheros and Ana de Zaballa Beascoechea, eds., *Los indios ante los foros de justicia religiosa en la hispanoamérica virreinal* (Mexico City, 2010); Kimberly Lynn, *Between Court and Confessional: The Politics of Spanish Inquisitors* (Cambridge, 2013); and John Chuchiak, ed., *The Inquisition in New Spain, 1536-1820: A Documentary History* (Baltimore, MD, 2012).

primitive or folk medicine.[11] New work in colonial Latin American history and the early modern Iberian world has begun to document the contribution of indigenous, African and other medical knowledges and practices to New World medical cultures.[12] Beneath these colonial discourses European, Mesoamerican and African medicine co-existed and intertwined in complicated and creative ways. There are few indigenous voices in the sources, however, which speak directly to the operation and extent of Mesoamerican medical cultures under Spanish colonial rule. Those sources that do contain first-hand reports and descriptions are often located within documents generated by the criminal and religious prosecution of Maya medical specialists, who somehow became tangled up in the institutional grasp of the Church, local authorities, or the Inquisition. We also find accounts of indigenous healers being consulted by the multi-ethnic sick and their families, Spanish elites and European travelers, all groups that utilized them. In contrast, there are few first-person narratives produced by the indigenous medical specialists themselves.

A close reading of the historical records, however, reveals the rough contours of robust, identifiably Mesoamerican medicinal cultures with distinct types of medical specialties practiced by indigenous women and men. I use the phrase 'Mesoamerican medical cultures' specifically to indicate that there was not one culture of Mesoamerican or indigenous medicine, but overlapping practices that varied by Maya ethnic group and by environment, and which influenced both illnesses that people in that area succumbed to, and the local geographic and cultural-based knowledge of plant, herbal and animal-based medicaments that mediated disease symptoms or offered cures.[13] Mesoameri-

---

11   The work of David Wade Chambers and Richard Gillespie, "Locality in the History of Science: Colonial Science, Technoscience, and Indigenous Knowledge," *Osiris*, 15 (2000), 221-240 was influential to my conceptualization of this issue. Scholars have recently begun take other medical cultures in the Americas seriously. See for example, Joan Bristol, *Christians, Blasphemers, and Witches: Afro-Mexican Ritual Practice in the Seventeenth Century* (Albuquerque, NM, 2007); Ryan Kashanipour, *Between Magic and Medicine: Colonial Yucatec Healing and the Spanish Atlantic World*, forthcoming from Omohundro Institute/ University of North Carolina Press, and his Ph.D. dissertation "A World of Cures: Yucatec Healing in the Eighteenth-Century Atlantic World" (University of Arizona, 2012); Martha Few, *For All of Humanity: Mesoamerican and Colonial Medicine in Enlightenment Guatemala* (Tucson, AZ, 2015); Pablo F. Gómez, *The Experiential Caribbean: Creating Knowledge and Healing in the Early Modern Atlantic* (Raleigh, NC, 2017), and Londa Schiebinger, *Secret Cures of Slaves: People, Plants, and Medicine in the Eighteenth-Century Atlantic World* (Stanford, CA, 2017).

12   See also Few, *For All of Humanity.*

13   Where possible I try and distinguish among these medical cultures, but often the sources available do not allow me to make such fine-grained distinctions.

can healers plied their trade within the scene of heterogeneous New World medical cultures that operated in Central America towards the end of the colonial period and beyond. Thus, this case study is important both because of the Inquisition's focus on rooting out a cross-cultural network of female ritual specialists in the initial years after the transition to a professional Inquisition in Spanish America, and because the illness treated – *mollera caída*, or fallen fontanel – provides one of the few archival examples from the colonial period of a culture specific illness still not fully understood by public health medicine today.

Accounts of ritual healing practices in colonial Central America like those used by Atichivalan and Atixiguite in Inquisition sources, however, were structured through the bureaucratic procedures and practices of the Holy Office. These are historical sources from a Spanish colonial institution, with roots in experiences in post-Reconquista royal state building efforts. Pope Sixtus IV had granted Queen Isabella and King Ferdinand the right to set up the Holy Office of the Inquisition in the territories they controlled (in Castile in 1478, and in Aragón in 1481), and the first tribunals of the Inquisition began there in 1482. Starting in 1532 in the Viceroyalty of New Spain, the Inquisition was run by members of the missionary orders and by the bishop of Mexico, and targeted mainly the newly converted indigenous populations. During the informal Inquisition era, however, many in Spain and New Spain found the punishments meted out to native peoples too harsh.[14]

To rebalance these excesses, the Crown established the formal Holy Office of the Inquisition in Spanish America in 1571, and set up a bureaucracy of Inquisitors, with its positions filled by men from Spain. Now the Inquisition in New Spain targeted members of all ethnic and social groups except indigenous peoples. Officially the Inquisition could no longer prosecute native peoples for religious crimes; that was supposed to fall to a parallel institution called the *Proviserato*. However, native peoples could still be called in as witnesses in Inquisition cases. With this transition, the highest Inquisition court in New Spain was now located in Mexico City, with Inquisition sub-courts located in the viceroyalties in major cities. In 1572 the Inquisition was formally established in Santiago de Guatemala. Officials investigated a wide range of complaints about religious crimes: heresy and apostasy, witchcraft and sorcery, pacts with the devil, bigamy and concubinage (especially among Spanish elites), solicitations in the confessional, blasphemy and the possession of prohibited books.

It was not until the 1650s that Inquisitional activity in colonial Guatemala primarily focused on more mundane crimes, and especially on what officials

---

14   See note 12.

characterized as sorcery. It did so largely in the capital city and surrounding small towns in the valley, rarely venturing further afield to places like Samayaq. Moreover, it was not until the mid-seventeenth century that the Inquisition targeted mixed-race and free Black populations, as well as women from these groups. This shift in emphasis coincided with the emergence of a multi-ethnic population in the capital city by the mid-seventeenth century: 60% of the total population of 39,000 was of mixed race, free and enslaved Blacks and non-tributary Indians.[15] With this significant mixed-race population in the capital, the Inquisition began to crack down on illegal religious activities and mundane crimes in the capital as one aspect of social control.[16]

Thus the Inquisition's investigation of the ritual activities of the healers of the Samayaq area is important both because of its focus on a cross-cultural network of female ritual specialists in the early years after the transition to a professional Inquisition, and because Inquisition officials in Santiago de Guatemala sanctioned the prosecution of indigenous women as part of the proceedings. By law, officials should have referred cases of accused indigenous men and women to other colonial bodies, such as ecclesiastical or civil courts and the *Proviserato*. In practice, however, the institutions had some overlap in policing indigenous religions deemed outside the bounds of Catholicism. Native peoples were frequently denounced to the Inquisition, but in most instances as soon as Inquisition authorities confirmed their legal status as Indian, those cases were then referred to these other colonial institutions.[17]

In the Samayaq investigation, all five accused indigenous women had the same *defensor* (a man named Pedro Rendero) assigned to them, a type of council for the defense that was required because of their legal standing as Indian (*india/o*) in colonial courts. Additionally many of those questioned only spoke indigenous languages. The court hired interpreters who had the ability to speak and understand the three languages used in the area, Spanish, Nahuatl (called in the documents *mexicana*) and Kaqchikel Maya (called in the documents *lengua materna*).[18] Padre Alonso Gutiérrez, who led the investigation in

---

15   The information in this paragraph is based on Christopher H. Lutz, *Santiago de Guatemala: City, Caste, and the Colonial Experience* (Norman, OK, 1994), 106-108, and Martha Few, *Women Who Live Evil Lives: Gender, Religion, and the Politics of Power in Colonial Guatemala* (Austin, TX, 2002), 20-23.

16   The majority of the Guatemalan Inquisition records are housed in the Archivo General de la Nación (AGN) in Mexico City.

17   Ernesto Chinchilla Aguilar, *La Inquisición en Guatemala* (Guatemala City, 1953), 25, 33; Few, *Women Who Live Evil Lives*, 28-30.

18   For the determination that Samayaq was a Kaqchikel-speaking town in the colonial period, see Francis Gall, *Diccionario geográfico de Guatemala* (Guatemala City, 1980), 3, 180. For a fascinating case study of two bigamy cases in this same region in the late

Samayaq, confined his questioning of witnesses to the families, neighbors and community members of the healers. There is no record that he questioned Alonso's mother, Doña María Velásquez, an elite Spanish woman married to the son of the town's *encomendera*, Juana López de Monzón. As encomendera, López de Monzón held the rights to tribute and labor from the indigenous residents of that town, called an *encomienda*.[19] Gutiérrez also did not question any other Spanish elites over the course of the case.

Fallen fontanel is today considered a 'culture specific' or 'folk' illness found in the Mesoamerican region. Other culture specific illnesses among people who lived in Mesoamerica and their descendants include *susto* (fright or soul loss) and *empacho* (obstructed stomach).[20] From the mid- to late twentieth century, there was some debate in medical anthropology research about whether fallen fontanel's origins as a disease category came from Spanish or Mesoamerican medical cultures. At root were disputes between those who depicted Mesoamerican medicine as derivative of Spanish professional and/or folk medicine, and those who argued that pre-Columbian Mesoamerican medical cultures were well developed and sophisticated. Proponents of this latter view thus characterized medicine practiced in colonial Latin America historically as syncretic, that is, as containing both Mesoamerican and European medical conceptions of disease and treatment methodologies, but arguing that the Mesoamerica strain was more influential or foundational and not simply derivative.[21]

---

sixteenth century, see Laura E. Matthew, "Two Bigamists in Tehuantepec: Globalization and Spatial Stories-So-Far, c. 1600," forthcoming. I thank her for graciously sharing her manuscript draft with me and for her helpful discussions about the Inquisition.

19   Doña María's Velaásquez's husband's name was Juan López de Monzón. Both are referred to by name in the Inquisition documents, as was Juana López de Monzón, the *encomendera* and likely widowed head of household.

20   See for example, Cevando Martínez and Harry W. Martin, "Folk Diseases among Urban Mexican-Americans," *Journal of the American Medical Association*, 196 (1966), 161-164; Joe S. Graham, "The Role of *Curanderos* in the Mexican-American Folk System in West Texas," in Wayland D. Hand, ed., *American Folk Medicine* (Berkeley, CA, 1976), 175-189; Byrd Howell Granger, "Some Aspects of Folk Medicine among Spanish-Speaking People in Southern Arizona," in Hand, ed., *American Folk Medicine*, 191-202; William R. Holland, "Mexican-American Medical Beliefs: Science or Magic?," in Ricardo Arguijo Martínez, ed., *Hispanic Culture and Health Care: Fact, Fiction, Folklore* (St. Louis, MS, 1978), 99-119; Susan C. Weller, Trenton K. Ruebush II and Robert E. Klein, "An Epidemiological Description of a Folk Illness: A Study of Empacho in Guatemala," *Medical Anthropology*, 13 (1991), 19-31; Susan C. Weller *et al.*, "Empacho in Four Latino Groups: A Study of Intra- and Inter- Cultural Variation in Beliefs," *Medical Anthropology*, 15 (1993), 109-136.

21   The foundational research that began these debates comes from the work of George Foster, starting with his journal article "Relationships between Spanish and Spanish

From our twenty-first century perspective it might not seem important that the sources used in this case study provide evidence of fallen fontanel, yet it is exceptional to find this particular illness, its diagnosis and descriptions of its treatment among a multi-ethnic population living in rural sixteenth-century Guatemala. It is also important because, in contemporary public health, doctors, nurses and others who treat immigrant populations in the United States from these regions, especially in the Southwest, continue to debate the boundaries of fallen fontanel as an illness category, as well as its causes and treatments.[22]

The testimonies recorded in the Inquisition sources repeatedly referred to fallen fontanel as something that everyone involved understood as an illness category, suggesting a broad and cross-cultural familiarity with the disease. Nowhere in the thirty-three folios that make up the case does anyone describe its symptoms. The sources do, however, provide eyewitness accounts of the healing strategies used to treat the disease, though filtered through the Inquisition investigation and the records drawn up by the notary in the third person.[23] Even so, there are points of agreement across the testimonies about what was

---

American Folk Medicine," *Journal of American Folklore*, 66 (1953), 201-217 along with supporters such as Margarita Kay in "The *Florilegio Medicinal:* Source of Southwest Ethnomedicine," *Ethnohistory*, 24 (1977), 251-259. For those who argue for sophisticated ancient Mesoamerican medical cultures and for fallen fontanel as an 'Aztec' illness category, see especially the work of Bernardo de Ortiz de Montellano, "Aztec Sources for a Mesoamerican Disease of Alleged Spanish Origin," *Ethnohistory*, 34 (1987), 381-399, and his monograph *Aztec Medicine, Health, and Nutrition* (New Brunswick, NJ, 1990). Ortiz de Montellano concludes that fallen fontanel is a disease that is "a syncretic mix of both native and European concepts, and in the case of *caída*, the pre-Columbian aspect predominates." Ortiz de Montellano, "Aztec Sources," 383.

22   See, for example, John Guarnaschelli, John Lee and Frederick W. Pitts, "Fallen Fontanelle (Caída de Mollera): A Variant of the Battered Child Syndrome," *Journal of the American Medical Association*, 222 (1972), 1545-1546; Robert T. Trotter II, Bernard Ortiz de Montellano and Michael H. Hogan, "Fallen Fontanelle in the American Southwest: Its Origin, Epidemiology, and Possible Organic Causes," *Medical Anthropology*, 10 (1989), 211-221; Anna Cornelia Gorter *et al.*, "Diarrea infantil en la Nicaragua rural: Creencias y prácticas de salud tradicional," *Boletín Oficina Sanitaria Panamericano*, 119 (1995), 377-390; Lee M. Pachter *et al.*, "Culture and Dehydration: A Comparative Study of Caída de la Mollera (Fallen Fontanel) in Three Latino Populations," *Journal of Immigrant and Minority Health*, 18 (2016), 1066-1075.

23   Testimonies written down in the documents are not a word-for-word transcription of what each person testified to. Instead they are likely a detailed summary and/or paraphrase of what was said, drafted first in notes and then formally written out by the notary according to legal protocols for these types of religious documents.

done in what order, evidence that indicates some shared understanding that the proper treatment necessitated a combination of divination, incantations, and the physical manipulation of the body. The wet nurse Catalina Sánchez witnessed both Atichivalan and Atixiguite treat Alonso at two different points in his illness. When Atichivalan arrived to the house to treat the infant, Isabel de Abrego pleaded with her to heal the boy. She consented after Abrego "took her by the hand."[24] Abrego's multiple requests, along with touching the healer as she asked a second time, show respect and demonstrate her recognition of Atichivalan's power as a healer. Atichivalan then took the boy into her arms and sat in a chair where she stretched out his legs and massaged his feet and toes. Next, she put her hand in the boy's mouth and blew a strong breath into it.[25] Then she lowered her hand and placed it on his feet; this she did twice. Finally, the healer opened her mouth and "exhaled a strong breath of air into the crown of the boy's head, using much force."[26] The boy's mother paid her two *reales,* a small amount of money at the time, and a gave her a cup of wine to drink.

Sánchez's description of the way Atixiguite treated fallen fontanel again began with repeated requests to get the healer to consent. Atixiguite relented, took the boy into her arms and sat on a *petate,* an indigenous-style mat woven from plant leaves. There she massaged the boy's toes, then put her hand in the infant's mouth and "*tomar el baho.*" The use of the verb "tomar" – 'to take' – here seems to indicate that Atixiguite sucked air out of his mouth, rather than blowing air into it. She then lowered her hands and massaged the feet and toes. Sánchez noted that both women spoke incantations or prayers during the ritual, but Sánchez did not understand what they said.[27] Doña María paid Atixiguite one *real* for her services. The fourteen-year old witness Magdalena Santiago, who watched Atixiguite treat a relative's daughter for fallen fontanel, remembered that the healer used divination. But because she had been young when the event had occurred a few years earlier, she did not remember any specific details.[28]

Doña Catalina Azetzun, an elite indigenous woman from the nearby small town of Chuliman, testified in Nahuatl through the official interpreter, and described how a woman named Chiquirincoa, also from Chuliman, treated the

---

24   "[T]omo la mano," AGN, Inq. vol. 209, exp. 2, f. 3r.
25   Ibid., f. 3v.
26   "[L]e echava vaho con ella en la mollera al niño haciendo para ello mucha ffuerça," ibid., ff. 1-33: ff. 3v-4r.
27   Ibid., f. 4r.
28   Ibid., f. 5r.

mulata María de Abrego's son Francisco for fallen fontanel.[29] Chiquirincoa followed a similar sequence of treatments: first she took the sick infant and massaged and manipulated his feet and toes. Next she put her hand in the boy's mouth to open it and then "exhaled a breath into his mouth and released humid air that rises."[30] This seems to indicate that this humid breath would work its way up through the mouth to raise the fontanel. Chiquirincoa repeated these steps four times, while saying a "prayer and other words" in Kaqchikel, incantations that Azetzun could not understand.[31]

Though in this Inquisition case colonial officials focused on Mesoamerican and multi-ethnic ritual medical methods of treating infants for fallen fontanel and other illnesses, the medical aspect of the case did not take center stage. No Spanish doctors were called in as expert witnesses in this case, nor did Inquisition officials ask them to offer explanations for fallen fontanel or medically treating infants in general. Anecdotal evidence for colonial Central America shows that medical physicians do not regularly appear in legal cases as expert witnesses in any consistent way until the eighteenth century. An exception is the role of female midwives who provided physical examinations and expert testimonies starting in the seventeenth century in cases of what we would today call rape and incest.[32]

Instead, the concern, as shown in the questions asked by Padre Gutiérrez as head of the local investigation and in his correspondence with regional political officials as well as diocesan bureaucrats in the capital, focused on the ritual aspects, and specifically on divination. Part of the reason for this emphasis had to do with the state of formal medicine in New Spain in general, and in colonial Central America specifically. The regulation of medical practice in New Spain and the *Audiencia* of Guatemala closely followed the Spanish model. In 1477 the Crown established the *Protomedicato*, an institution designed to regulate medicine through examinations, licensing and the court system. The Spanish crown continued this institution in New Spain, and in 1525 the municipal council of Mexico City named its first *Protomédico*, to regulate medical practices there. The *Protomedicato* did not license Muslim or Jewish doctors, nor did it license native healers.

---

29 Ibid., ff. 6r-7r. I infer that Azetzun is a Nahuatl speaker, because in her testimony she revealed that she could not understand the Kaqchikel that the curers used when they treated the infant. Furthermore I judge that Francisco was sick with fallen fontanel, even though Azetzun vaguely refers to his symptoms as "certain sicknesses," because the description is similar to Catalina Sanchez's account above.

30 Ibid., f. 6v.

31 Ibid.

32 See Few, *For All of Humanity*, 96-132.

For much of the colonial period, however, especially outside of urban centers, formal medical presence and the reach of the *Protomedicato* was minimal to non-existent. Guatemala's university, the Universidad de San Carlos, which included a medical school, was not established until 1680.[33] There was a chronic shortage of licensed physicians in colonial Guatemala, and this can be seen, in part, by repeated requests from Santiago de Guatemala's city council asking Mexico City's city council to send a licensed medical doctor to the capital, along with repeated attempts to raise funds among local elites to ensure that the salary would attract and keep the doctor in the capital.[34] There were four hospitals in late sixteenth-century Guatemala, and each cared for a specific sector of the population: The Royal Hospital of Santiago was established in 1541 by Bishop Francisco Marroquín; it only treated Spaniards. Construction was completed in 1553.[35] The Hospital San Alejo exclusively treated indigenous people; the Hospital San Pedro tended to priests; and the Hospital San Lázaro cared for those with leprosy and other diseases deemed infectious.[36] For the most part, however, those living in colonial Central America devised multiple healing strategies that included some combination of consulting professional medical doctors, practically trained barber-surgeons, native healers, Black and multi-ethnic *curanderos* and midwives, the use of home remedies and pilgrimages to healing shrines.[37]

Another reason for the Inquisition's emphasis on policing the supernatural, and more precisely divinatory aspects of the women's healing activities had to do with the fact that it had only been fifty years, more or less, since the conquest period. For central Mexico, historians mark the end of the conquest period with the decisive military defeat of the Aztec/Mexica capital city Tenochtitlan (today's Mexico City) in 1521. In contrast, the conquest period in

33   For an introduction to the early history of medicine and medical practice in colonial New Spain, see John Tate Lanning, *The Royal Protomedicato: The Regulation of the Medical Professions in the Spanish Empire*, ed. John TePaske (Durham, 1985), and Guenter B. Risse, "Medicine in New Spain," in Ronald L. Numbers, ed., *Medicine in the New World: New Spain, New France, and New England* (Knoxville, TN, 1987), 12-63.

34   J. Joaquín Pardo, *Efemerides para escribir la historia de la muy noble y muy leal ciudad de Santiago de los Caballeros del Reino de Guatemala* (Guatemala City, 1944), *passim*.

35   Julio Roberto Herrera, "Anotaciones y documentos para la historia de los hospitales de la ciudad de Santiago de los Caballeros de Guatemala," *Anales de la Sociedad de Geografía e Historia*, 8 (1942), 225-272.

36   Ibid., 228, 231.

37   The use of combinations of medical paradigms is common today, including in the United States. For more on local healers in colonial New Spain, see the work of Noemí Quezada, especially *Enfermedad y maleficio: El curandero en el México colonial* (Mexico City, 1989).

Central America, especially in the Guatemalan highlands, dragged on, as this area contained a number of Maya city-states that each needed to be militarily defeated by Spanish forces and their indigenous allies from central Mexico: the K'iche', Kaqchikel, M'am, Tzutuhil and other Maya ethnic groups.[38] The last independent Maya kingdom of the Itza' Maya, located in what is now the Petén region of modern Guatemala, was not defeated by Spanish colonial forces until the late 1690s.[39] And so we find in this case of the prosecution of 'divination' and 'sorcery' the fascinating outlines of an extensive, informal multi-ethnic network of female ritual-medical specialists who practiced their trades in and around Samayaq – a network that even the most important Spanish family in town drew on when their infant son became ill with fallen fontanel.

But why should Inquisition officials concern themselves with Samayaq, a small, seemingly inconsequential town in an *Audiencia* on the edge of empire? Clues lie in the history of the town itself and its roots as an important religious center that spanned the pre-conquest and colonial eras. In the Postclassic era (c. 900-1521) the town was known as Tzaamayac and acted as the seat of Tzutuhil and K'iche' Maya *sacerdotes*, 'priests' or ritual specialists.[40] In the sixteenth century, Spanish colonial officials renamed the town San Francisco Samayaq. The town retained its reputation as a religious center under colonial rule as well, when, by the 1570s and around the time of this Inquisition investigation, it became the site of a Franciscan monastery with a supporting tributary Indian population of 450 persons.[41] There, however, the town's Mesoamerican religious-ritual cultures adapted and endured through the colonial period. When Archbishop Pedro Cortés y Larraz made his 1769-1770 inspection of the towns in his jurisdiction across colonial Central America, Samayaq's parish priest spoke to him of active indigenous ritual practices there, conducted at night by the town's "fortune tellers, healers, and evil-doers" in "the mountains" (*los montes*).[42] The priest also mentioned the existence a *calendario* or *almanak*, an indigenous language ritual book "that they [the indigenous leaders of Samayaq] use for their governance."[43] Cortés y Larraz described himself horrified to hear of the existence of such a ritual book "that they use in all the

---

38   A good, general introduction to the protracted conquest period in the Maya areas of what is now Central America and Mexico can be found in Robert M. Carmack, *The Legacy of Mesoamerica: History and Culture of a Native American Civilization* (New York, NY, 1995).

39   See Grant D. Jones, *Conquest of the Last Maya Kingdom* (Stanford, CA, 1998).

40   Gall, *Diccionario geográfico*, vol. 3, 178.

41   Ibid., 179.

42   Pedro Cortés y Larraz, *Descripción geográfico-moral de la Diocesis de Goathemal*, 2 vols. (Guatemala City, 1958), vol. 2, 156: "[A]goreros, curanderos y maleficos."

43   Ibid., 157.

Kaqchikel, K'iche', and Mam [Maya] parishes, and it is the same [here], though written in their own language."[44]

Public displays of the ritual power of colonial Christianity to halt illness and epidemics in times of community stress comprised part of the broader ideological labor performed by priests and Church officials in Latin America that helped legitimate the ideology of colonial rule. Priests, acting as ritual specialists, led religious processions, public ceremonies and rites during epidemics, drought, flooding, locust plagues and earthquakes, all of which were part of life in colonial Guatemala.[45] Religious officials also displayed the power of colonial Christianity to mediate mundane aspects of illness and death as well. Priests regularly made judgments about the time when death was likely to occur in the sick and elderly, so that they could administer death rites and rituals.[46]

Of course colonial Christianity did not monopolize the use of ritual power in the face of epidemics and illness, and priests were not the only persons to predict times of death. In Postclassic and colonial Maya cultures, medicine and religious practice tied together in ritual activities designed to address matters of illness and death, and these continued to operate after the consolidation of Spanish rule. An important part of colonial Mesoamerican ritual cultures involved the divination that allowed a Maya healer to make informed judgments of whether the sick would recover or die from an illness, whether or not an epidemic was immanent, and to ensure community protection from, and the expulsion of, epidemic diseases.[47] With the arrival of European colonialism, Mesoamerican medical cultures flexibly adjusted to adapt and create medico-religious responses to new epidemic diseases such as smallpox and other illnesses into their ritual-medical array.

How did colonial political officials, priests and town residents know ritual practices of indigenous medicine when they saw them, and what can we infer from this case about the reasons why they considered the women's activities

---

44   Here I have updated the spelling of the Maya ethnic groups. "Que éste es el almanak de que se usa en todas las parroquias del kacchiquel y kiché, y en el mam, es el mismo, pero escrito en su propio idioma," ibid., 156.

45   I deliberately use the phrase 'ritual specialist' to describe both Spanish priests and Maya healers as being concerned with what we would today call 'religious labor' and 'medical labor' in public and private displays of their specialized power, even though they themselves did not make a distinction between the two.

46   This was a matter of competition and conflict with learned physicians as well. For more on the rituals used by priests to determine the time of death, see Francisco Xavier Lascano, *Indice práctico-moral para los sacerdotes que auxilian moribundos* (Guatemala, 1754).

47   The Spanish verb used in the sources to refer to this activity is *adivinar*.

dangerous? Right from the start, the judge provisor Don Francisco González linked divination (*adivinas*) to sorcery (*sortilegas*) in characterizing what Atichivalan and Atixiguite used when treating Alonso and other infants with fallen fontanel in the area. González highlighted, in particular, their activities of "making supplications and prayers, tossing certain things over hot coals, speaking with the fire, and rapidly massaging the toes."[48] Here, he connected the speech acts of incantations and communication with the fire and the smell from the burning of certain undescribed materials. This ritual act provided the information that the healer needed to know where and how to touch and manipulate the sick body. To fourteen-year-old Magdalena de Santiago, Atixiguite's divination with fire was the integral part of her description of the woman's treatment of an infant girl for fallen fontanel a few years earlier.[49] According to Santiago, Atixiguite asked the others present to bring her some hot coals in a piece of pottery, and then she threw some small sticks and herbs into the fire that she built with the coals.[50] She could not describe any subsequent details of the ritual healing, saying that she "did not understand what happened" to the infant.[51]

Many of those questioned in the case spoke of the two Maya curers as having a regional reputation for their healing skills. Furthermore, most of the witnesses referred to the women by their Kaqchikel names, and not by their Hispanicized or the formal names recorded by the notary. Magdalena de Santiago, for example, referred to "the old female healer whose name in their maternal language is Atixiguite," with a reputation as someone who "knows how to cure sickness."[52] The witness Doña Catalina Azetzun, the married indigenous resident of the Chuliman, added two more women to the list of local ritual specialists who used divination to treat infants and children, a woman called Chiquirincoa and the wife of Martín Hune, whose name she could not remember. Both lived in her small town and had reputations as ritual specialists, as did Atichivalan and Atixiguite, she said, adding that all four women practiced divination.[53]

Mesoamerican ritual cultures also included divination using a variety of methods to determine whether a sick person would recover or die from their

---

48   AGN, Inq. vol. 209, exp. 2, f. 1v.

49   Ibid., f. 4v. Magdalena de Santiago was the daughter of Francisco de Santiago. She was listed as *soltera* (unmarried) and *doncella* (an unmarried virgin, and thus honorable).

50   Ibid., f. 4v.

51   "[E]sta testigo nunca entendio lo que desto ," ibid., f. 5r.

52   Ibid., ff. 4v- 5r.

53   Ibid., f. 5v.

illness, yet we see this practice referred to only in vague terms by the witnesses questioned in this case. What seemed to matter, or at least what individuals decided to tell the authorities, was whether the ritual specialist prophesied death or not. The wet nurse Catalina Sánchez provided a little information on how Atixiguite prophesied that Alonso would die from the illness: "And the old woman took the boy and touched him (*tentar*), and placed her hand on top of his head," and then predicted that Alonso would die.[54] This description may refer to some type of laying on of hands, as practiced in both Christian and Mesoamerican ritual-medical strategies.[55]

What made the divination practiced by the women suspicious was the witnesses's inability to understand the words in incantations and prayers uttered by the healers as they treated sick infants. Isabel de la Cerda, who was married to the local merchant trader Gaspar de la Feria, told the authorities that Chiquirincoa was an *adivina* (a divination specialist) who knew how to divine whether a sick person would recover or die, who could describe the details of the lives of loved ones who had migrated permanently or seasonally to other towns, and who had the ability to locate missing belongings and domestic animals including, in one case, a lost horse.[56] De la Cerda had heard from a friend of her husband's about the ritual-medical practices used to treat Alonso's fallen fontanel, that "one of the old Indian women" (she was not sure who) "took the boy and did certain things to him, crying out, and transforming her face into a demon's face."[57] This combination of words and 'cries' that other community members could not understand, and strange, demon-like faces that transformed the healer during the divination, runs through the testimonies that made the women's actions suspicious.

As Padre Gutiérrez, the appointed judge from San Antonio Suchitepéquez, and the notary heard and recorded testimonies, they hired two court interpreters to assist with the case. Francisco Ximénez was described as an *yndio ladino* (lit. 'ladino Indian'; a Hispanicized indigenous man), a resident of the area who understood and spoke "the Mexican language, Castilian and the maternal lan-

---

54   "[Y] la dicha vieja tomo el niño e lo tento poniendole la mano encima," ibid., f. 4r.

55   For more on ancient Mesoamerican understandings of the human body, illness and healing see for example Alfredo López Austin, *The Human Body and Ideology: Concepts of the Ancient Nahuas*, 2 vols, trans. Thelma Ortiz de Montellano and Bernard Ortiz de Montellano (Salt Lake City, UT, 1980), and Bernard R. Ortiz de Montellano, *Aztec Medicine, Health, and Nutrition* (New Brunswick, NJ, 1990).

56   AGN, Inq. vol. 209, exp. 2, f. 20v.

57   "[Q]ue avia tomado [una vieja india] el niño e hecho ciertas cosas y dado gritos, e puestosele la cara como la del demonio," ibid., f. 8r-v.

guage of the indigenous people of this [Pacific] coast."[58] Agustín Pérez, also a ladino Indian with the same linguistic skills, took over at times when Ximénez was not available.[59] Pérez's interpreter role was particularly important once the arrest orders went out in March of 1695; he accompanied the men sent to arrest the women as they only spoke indigenous languages. Pérez also accompanied officials who followed up on the arrests by confiscating the women's properties. Each of the five of the indigenous women testified in indigenous languages with the help of the interpreter Ximénez.[60]

These legal proceedings had begun on 29 February 1596. A little less than three weeks later, by 16 March, Padre Gutiérrez felt that he had enough information to take the next set of steps against the seven women and he signed an *auto de prison*, a judicial decree that ordered their arrest.[61] This decree did not go through the formal Inquisition in Santiago de Guatemala; instead, Padre Gutiérrez requested and received legal permission from don Vasco de Guzmán, the *alcalde mayor* of the province Zapotitlán y Suchitépequez, because the town of Samayaq lay in this political jurisdiction.[62] Once arrested, the women were housed by the officials in the episcopal jail (*carcel episcopal*) which was located in San Antonio Suchitepéquez, except for Isabel de Abrego, who was not home when the officials arrived and was thought to have fled. Interestingly, because of the translators working on the case and even with a professional notary keeping records, Gutiérrez's official order only identified Isabel de Abrego and María de Abrego by their correct, full names. He either mangled the names, provided partial names, or gave only the husbands' names to identify five indigenous women to be arrested: "[the] *fulanas* (lit. "the so and sos") Tichivalan and Anziguite and Chiquirincoa and the wife of Martín Hene and the wife of Diego Juanha."[63] That same judicial decree gave Gutiérrez the permission to seize the accused indigenous women's possessions, including their houses, the fruits of their agricultural lands and their material goods (Isabel and María Abrego's possessions, however, were not confiscated). It is unclear whether Gutiérrez did this to look for illegal ritual items, or to simply increase the intimidation campaign that would eventually lead to the women's confessional proceedings.[64]

---

58 Ibid., ff. 2r and 10v.
59 Ibid., f. 1v.
60 The *confessiones* for all seven women, including the Isabel Abrego and María Abrego, begin on folio 17v of the proceedings.
61 Ibid., f. 15v.
62 Ibid.
63 Ibid., f. 16r.
64 Ibid., f. 15v.

Three days later, on 19 March, Gutiérrez brought each of the indigenous women to the makeshift religious court to take their confessions. He questioned them closely, through interpreter Ximénez, on the charges of sorcery, divination and a host of other supernatural activities.[65] Also present was the women's court-appointed lawyer, Pedro Rendón. None of the five women confessed to any illegal activity; most denied even knowing each other, despite the fact that they lived in Samayaq or nearby small villages.

Isabel Chivalan (alias Atichivalan) was a widow who did not know her age, though the notary judged her to be more that 70 years old. She told the court that she did not know Isabel de Abrego or her adult daughter María. When asked directly if she was a sorcerer (*hechicera*) who used "words of enchantment and superstitions" to cure people, she denied it.[66] Isabel Roche Guigir (alias Atixiguite) was married. She also did not know her exact age, but she seemed to colonial officials to be about fifty years old. Atixiguite knew Atichivalan and María de Abrego, but denied treating Alonso for fallen fontanel, summing up that "she [Atiguite] is a midwife (*partera*) in this town, and has no other trade other than this with which to earn a living."[67] Catalina Hune, who was also married, appeared to be more than fifty years old. Gutierréz asked her if she was a "witch and a sorcerer who uses enchanted words for whatever Indian man or woman is sick in the town of Samayaq, causing a notable scandal and serving as a bad example to other Indians," but she denied it, and claimed that she did not know the Abregos. Furthermore, Hune refuted the contention that she used sorcery, and concluded that she was "a good Christian, fearful of God in her body and soul."[68]

Catalina Chirincoa was the last of the imprisoned indigenous healers to be questioned. She, too, spoke through the interpreter, appeared to be about fifty years old, and was married. Chirincoa said that she knew the Abregos, but refused to admit that she practiced sorcery.[69] Gutiérrez questioned the married woman Isabel Juaniha last, who was thought to be more than sixty years old and also spoke through the interpreter.[70] Juaniha claimed that she did not

---

65   Ibid., f. 22r.
66   "[P]or palabras de encantamiento y supersticiones," ibid., f. 22v.
67   "Ffuele preguntado diga e declare si es verdad que esta confesante es hechicera y sortiliza e usa de palabras de encantamiento en el dicho pueblo de Çamayaque dando notable escandalo y mal exemplo a los naturales," and "y esta confesante tan solamente es partera en el dicho pueblo, y no tiene oficio mas deste en que gana su vida," ibid., f. 24r.
68   "[Y] esta confesante es buena christiana temerosa de Dios y de su conçiencia y persona," ibid., f. 25r.
69   Ibid., f. 26r.
70   Ibid., f. 27r.

know María and Isabel de Abrego, and that she was not a "sorcerer who uses divination" nor someone who "speaks words that no one understands."[71] After the confession phase finished, all five indigenous women had denied using sorcery or divination; only Isabel Roche Guigir (aka Atixiguite) admitted to practicing the medical arts as a midwife. The case ends there; we do not know anything further.

Midwives and healers who treated infants and children in late sixteenth-century Guatemala, and even to the present day, were both practical and religious specialists who mediated the natural and supernatural realms through divination. Casting herbs onto coals and 'speaking with the fire' was one method they used to interpret the signs on a child's body to make determinations about the cause of an illness, how to treat it and chances for survival. As guardians of maternal, infant and child health, these healers played socially critical roles, especially in sixteenth-century colonial Guatemala, where indigenous populations had suffered devastating population losses due to violence and especially epidemic disease. Community perceptions and rumors that the healers used supernatural means, including divination, to treat infants, including the son of the town's elite Spanish *encomendero* family, as well as the mixed-race child of María de Abrego and infants from other nearby pueblos, reflected continued experiences of suffering, illness and dislocation in rural Maya towns under Spanish rule, as well as an apprehension about women's roles as healers and ritual specialists in community life.

---

71   "[S]ortilega hechizera y usa de adivina" and "habla unas palabras que no se entienden," ibid., f. 27r-v.

Physicians and Surgeons in the Service of the Portuguese Inquisition: Twelve Years After

Timothy D. Walker
University of Massachusetts Dartmouth
twalker@umassd.edu

During the past quarter century, in part because of increased historiographical interest in the prosecution of witchcraft and other magical crimes (including superstitious folk healing) by European ecclesiastical authorities, scholars have begun to better understand the influential connections between religious institutions like the Holy Office of the Inquisition and the evolution of medicine, both as a field of knowledge and as a profession. Thus, the general focus of the present volume – medicine and the Inquisition in the early modern world – represents a logical epistemological progression of scholarly attention directed toward a more nuanced assessment of ways that inquisitors, physicians, and surgeons interacted, occasionally forming synergistic relationships in sixteenth- to eighteenth-century Europe. As this and the other chapters included in this volume demonstrate, exploring the intersection of these powerful social actors – the sometimes colliding, other times collaborating Holy Office and medical professionals – can result in rich insights about the various ways these players interacted, or exercised agency and influence, often disproportionate to their size or numbers of personnel, within the historical societies they occupied.

This chapter will focus on the role of physicians and surgeons who worked within the ranks of the Portuguese Inquisition to prosecute and discredit popular healers (called *saludadores* or *curandeiros*), who in eighteenth-century Portugal were tried under the centuries-old laws that condemned the practice of witchcraft and sorcery. It is a revised and updated version of a work originally published in 2007.[1] Looking back over the intervening twelve years, while

---

*   University of Massachusetts Dartmouth, 285 Old Westport Road, North Dartmouth, MA 02747, USA. twalker@umassd.edu

1   This is a revised and updated version of a chapter originally published in Ole Peter Grell and Andrew Cunningham, eds., *Medicine and Religion in Enlightenment Europe* (Farnham, 2007). I am grateful to the Taylor & Francis Group for their kind permission to use this material.

it is difficult to assess and comment retrospectively about the impact of that article after such a relatively short period of time, it appears that the original publication did play some historiographical role as a component in a diverse body of work that served as a catalyst for subsequent scholarship. Innovative, important work about the historical spaces where science, medicine, the Inquisition, and other religious organizations of the Iberian Peninsula intersected can be found in works published in the past decade by such scholars as James Sweet and Pablo Gomez, among others.[2] To these may be added the incisive new works produced here by Hervé Baudry, Alessandra Celati, Bradford A. Bouley and Maria Pia Donato. Taken together, this body of pioneering scholarship expands on and improves our understanding of the themes and circumstances explored in my article from twelve years ago, and points toward intriguing paths of research on the attitude of medical practitioners vis-à-vis both ecclesiastical power and popular culture.

•••

The most intense period of "witch-hunting" in Portugal (*circa* 1715-1760) corresponds exactly with the period in which Portuguese physicians and surgeons were becoming more aware of new medical techniques being developed outside of Portugal.[3] The period also coincides with a time in which licensed

I wish to thank the Instituto Camões, the United States Fulbright Commission, and the Council for International Educational Exchange for providing the grants that made this research possible. For logistical support in Lisbon, Portugal, I am grateful to the Arquivo Nacional do Torre do Tombo, the Biblioteca Nacional de Lisboa and the Academia des Ciências de Lisboa. The Wellcome Trust provided additional financial and academic support for this project, making possible additional research in London.

2   See, among others, Pablo F. Gómez, *The Experiential Caribbean: Creating Knowledge and Healing in the Early Modern Atlantic* (Chapel Hill, 2017); Matthew James Crawford, *The Andean Wonder Drug: Cinchona Bark and Imperial Science in the Spanish Atlantic, 1630-1800* (Pittsburgh, 2016); Benjamin Patrick Breen, "Empires on Drugs: Materia Medica and the Anglo-Portuguese Alliance," in Jorge Cañizares-Esguerra, ed., *Entangled Empires: The Anglo-Iberian Atlantic, 1500-1830* (Philadelphia, 2018); Marta Hanson and Gianna Pomata, "Medicinal Formulas and Experiential Knowledge in the Seventeenth-century Epistemic Exchange between China and Europe," *Isis* 108 (2017), 1-25; Hugh Cagle, *Assembling the Tropics: Science and Medicine in Portugal's Empire, 1450-1700* (Cambridge, 2018); James H. Sweet, *Domingos Alvares, African Healing, and the Intellectual History of the Atlantic World* (Chapel Hill, 2011); Daniel Norte Giebels, *A Inquisição de Lisboa: no epicentro da dinâmica inquisitorial (1537-1579)* (Ph.D. thesis, University of Coimbra, 2016).

3   Ana Carneiro, Ana Simões, and Maria Paula Diogo, "The Scientific Revolution in Eighteenth-century Portugal: The Role of the Estrangeirados (Europeanized Intellectuals)," *Social Studies of Science,* 30 (2000), 591-619, and "Constructing Knowledge: Eighteenth-century Portugal and the New Sciences," *Archimedes,* 2 (1999), 1-40.

medical professionals had become firmly ensconced in the ranks of the Holy Office in substantial numbers – particularly influential physicians and surgeons in Coimbra, the medieval university town that was home to Portugal's only faculty of medicine.[4] These circumstances are not mere coincidence. Indeed, the cadence of Inquisition trials for sorcery and witchcraft in Portugal increased dramatically at the end of the seventeenth century, reached a peak between 1715 and 1760, and dropped sharply after 1772. During this period, in approximately 60% of Holy Office trials in which the suspect was accused of a crime entailing the use of magic or superstitions, the culprit was actually a healer engaged in providing folk remedies to rural peasants and townspeople. Such cures relied on illicit acts of sorcery for their efficacy. These "witchcraft" cases reflect an increasing intolerance for folk healers among the previously indifferent inquisitors and other elites.

The proclivity of the Portuguese Inquisition to prosecute popular healers during the eighteenth century was the result of a deliberate policy on behalf of medical professionals inside the Inquisition who, in combination with their ecclesiastical colleagues, acted on their concurrent compatible vested interests to discredit popular medicine and its practitioners, with the eventual goal of eliminating superstitious folk healing from the Portuguese realm.

Significantly, the peak period of witchcraft persecution in Portugal coincided with a time when university-trained physicians and surgeons, or *médicos*, were entering the paid ranks of the Inquisition in unprecedented numbers, taking up employment as *familiares* (non-ecclesiastical employees of the Holy Office – informants who often identified deviant members of society as potential subjects for an Inquisition investigation) to enjoy the status and privileges consequent to holding such a post. State-licensed physicians and surgeons, motivated by professional competition but also by a concern for promoting scientific medicine, used their positions within the Holy Office to initiate trials against purveyors of superstitious folk remedies.

Thus, the persecution of *curandeiros* and *saludadores* reveals a conflict between learned medical culture and popular healing culture, as well as an alignment of interests between professional licensed healers and the Inquisition. This tension between popular culture and elite culture grew as the Enlightenment era advanced and rationalist ideas about medicine flowed into Portugal through unofficial channels (but frequently with the tacit consent of reactionary, orthodox state and Church officials). Holy Office trials against magical

---

4   José Viega Torres, "Da repressão religiosa para a promoção social: a Inquisição como instância legitimadora da promoção social da burguesia mercantil," *Revista crítica de ciências sociais*, 40 (1994), 109-135.

healers, then, offer evidence that Enlightenment ideas about rationalized medical practices had penetrated the minds of learned elites in Portugal to such a degree that even the policies of the Inquisition changed to accommodate, and even promote, a novel approach to healing. In this rare instance, the Inquisition arguably functioned as an instrument of progressive social change.

In terms of tone and intent, the Portuguese experience with prosecuting magical healing was unique in early modern Europe; Inquisition authorities brought over five hundred magical healers and sorcerers to trial between 1715 and 1770, but they did not execute a single one.[5] Although some regions across Europe continued to prosecute small numbers of "witches" throughout the eighteenth century, no country except Portugal experienced such a sizable and sustained incidence of trials, centrally directed according to an explicit rationalist policy, against magical criminals at such a late date. The chronology of magical crimes trials in Portugal, occurring as they did simultaneously with a demonstrable awakening of interest in scientific investigation and natural philosophy in that country, makes these cases particularly interesting for scholars of the confrontation between Enlightenment sensibilities and popular superstitions.

In other words, there was a conscious, deliberate and systematic movement by licensed *médicos* to discredit popular *curandeiros* and *saludadores* in the minds of common people and sow widespread doubt about traditional forms of healing. Further, in singling out popular healers for persecution, it is evident that many of these doctors were motivated by a genuine wish to effect rationalized scientific medical reforms; they were not simply trying to eliminate their professional competitors.

Continental Portugal was divided into three Holy Office districts, each with its own Inquisition tribunal, associated prison, and cadre of functionaries. The majority of Holy Office cases against *curandeiros* or *saludadores* originated with the Inquisition tribunal located in the city of Coimbra. Further, the Coimbra tribunal's rate of persecution of popular healers began to rise sharply well before the other two tribunals in Évora and Lisbon began to pursue *curandeiros* more actively. The Holy Office's movement of prosecuting illicit healers, then, began in Coimbra, Portugal's seat of academic medical training.[6]

---

5   José Pedro Paiva, *Bruxaria e superstição num país sem 'caça às bruxas': Portugal 1600-1774* (Lisbon, 1997), 209.

6   These assertions point to *curandeiro* trials conducted in Coimbra between 1710 and 1714, the half-decade immediately prior to the forty-year period identified as the peak years of Portuguese witch-hunting. While it is true that the Évora tribunal demonstrated a strong inclination to prosecute *mágicos*, too, during the same half-decade, 1710-1714, in none of those cases was the person tried a *curandeiro*. See tables following chapter VIII in Timothy D. Walker,

The Inquisition tribunal operating in Coimbra had, by the end of the seventeenth century, forged a profound and multi-faceted link with the faculty of medicine at the University of Coimbra, not only employing trained physicians and surgeons in the Holy Office prisons, but also using licensed professional medical practitioners widely as informants and functionaries. Several prominent instructors of the faculty of medicine were in fact Inquisition *familiares*, as were many of their then-current and former students.[7] Indeed, during the eighteenth century, the chief *médico* of the Inquisition prisons in Coimbra was also typically a Coimbra University professor of one of the medical disciplines.[8]

The University of Coimbra and its environs provided the place where licensed practitioners of medicine would become most conscious of themselves as a distinct professional and social group.[9] And yet, in this Jesuit-dominated institution where the basic structure and content of the medical curriculum had not changed in three centuries, forward-thinking physicians and surgeons found their desire for enlightened reform indefinitely stymied. By extension, then, it is logical that Coimbra would also be the location where medical practitioners would first come to see that popular healers constituted a threat to their collective professional endeavors.

Having already established a link with the Inquisition – the strength of which kept growing as more licensed physicians, surgeons and barbers became *familiares* – medical professionals possessed a means at their disposal to act against this threat. Later, as the eighteenth century progressed and more Portuguese physicians and surgeons became aware (and enamored) of the scientific techniques being practiced in other parts of Europe, they became motivated by more erudite reasons to discredit and drive out popular healers. Because Portuguese *médicos* were thwarted from instituting modern medical practices through the University of Coimbra, one of their only avenues to promote modernization lay in using the Inquisition to discredit popular healers, thereby advancing their case for the Enlightenment reform of healing practices.

Doctors, Folk Medicine and the Inquisition: The Repression of Magical Healing in Portugal during the Enlightenment (Leiden, 2005), 321-331.

7   Giuseppe Marcocci and José Pedro Paiva, *História da Inquisição portuguesa (1536-1821)* (Lisbon, 2013), 255-259, 296-298.

8   Walker, *Doctors*, 180-189.

9   Teophilo Braga, *História da Universidade de Coimbra*, (Lisbon, 1895), 2: 768-812. See also José Sebastião da Silva Dias, *Portugal e a cultura europeia: séculos XVI a XVIII* (Coimbra, 1952), 280-299; Rocha Brito e Feliciano Guimarães, "A Faculdade de Medicina de Coimbra," *Actas Ciba*, 14 (1950), 508-586.

The State of Medical Teaching at the University of Coimbra during the Eighteenth Century

Throughout the seventeenth and much of the eighteenth centuries, professors of medicine at the University of Coimbra were reduced to intoning rote, undeviating recitations and commentary on the writings of the ancient and medieval medical authorities: Galen, Hippocrates, Rhazes, and Avicenna. Even after the restoration of the Portuguese crown in 1640, when pedagogical modifications following a sixty-year period of Spanish influence might have been expected, the teaching curriculum in the *Faculdade de Medicina* remained, with very few changes, virtually as it had existed throughout the 1500s.

Until the enlightened autocratic Prime Minister Pombal's reforms of 1772 revitalized medical instruction at Coimbra, there was little in the way of practical hands-on training; medical lectures remained theoretical, as they had been for centuries. Even in the mid-eighteenth century, instructors performed human dissections extremely rarely (*rarissimamente*).[10] Bodies for educational dissection, when they could be obtained, usually had to be those of condemned criminals, preferably those of non-Catholics or known heretics. Some cadavers, no doubt, became available following an untimely death among those incarcerated for heretical crimes in the local Inquisition prison.

One eighteenth-century Portuguese medical reformer spoke out in apology for those who had to work within this archaic system. João Mendes Sachetti Barbosa, a doctor of the *Alentejo* province who corresponded with expatriate colleagues (*estrangeirados*) and would later help create the progressive Royal Medical Academy of Oporto (founded 1749), excused the reactionary teaching habits of his mentors at Coimbra, arguing in 1756 that "if they defend Galen and Avicenna," it was not because of their own inability or lack of better training, but instead because of a strict observance of the law and "reverential respect for its statutes."[11]

Parenthetically, Sachetti Barbosa was of Old Christian ancestry and, like many ambitious physicians of his day, he looked upon employment with the Holy Office as a means to greater status and opportunity in Portuguese society, particularly in the rural *Alentejo*. Following the path of his brother, António

---

10   Brito and Guimarães, "A Faculdade," 555-556; Maximiano José de Morais Correia, *Subsídios para a história da anatomía em Coimbra* (Coimbra, 1950).

11   João Mendes Sachetti Barbosa, *Considerações médicas doctrinais sobre a metodo conhecer, curar e preservar as epidemias, ou febras malignas podres, pestilenciaes e contagiozas* (Lisbon, 1758), xxvii. On the Oporto academy, see José Pedro Sousa Dias, "Equívocos sobre a ciência moderna nas academias médico-cirúrgicas portuenses," in *Medicamento, história e sociedade*, 1 (1992), 2-9.

Mendes Sachetti, who was the chief treasurer of the Cathedral at Elvas and a commissioner of the Inquisition tribunal of Évora, he applied to become a *familiar* of the Holy Office. Sachetti Barbosa received his letter appointing him an employee of the Inquisition on 12 March 1756.[12] Within two years, he had been named a physician of the Royal Household and a Knight and Peer of the *Casa Real*. In 1759, he was made a Knight of the Order of Christ, an extraordinarily prestigious honor for a rural physician of common stock. From humble beginnings, this reform-minded country doctor rapidly came to enjoy royal favor.[13] He was not alone: fellow Oporto Medical Academy founding member Manuel Freire da Paz, one of the directors of the Royal Hospital in Coimbra (his title was *Médico de relação e do Senado de Câmara*), a contender for a teaching post on the Faculty of Medicine, and future Knight of the Order of Christ (1751), had become a *familiar* of the Holy Office in Coimbra on 27 February 1743.[14] Even the Academy founder, Manuel Gomes de Lima, was a Holy Office *familiar*. Clearly, these university-trained physicians felt no contradiction that would prevent them from working for two institutions with such differing approaches to scientific innovation.

The Portuguese universities did of course harbor some men of science who did not share the prevailing conservative sentiments in the upper echelons of the Portuguese Church and state, but instructors still had to acquiesce to regulations set by the Jesuits governing what they could and could not teach. Maximiano Lemos, Portugal's preeminent historian of medicine, went as far as asserting that the state of medical science was more advanced outside the university setting, because of scientific treatises provided surreptitiously by *converso* or Jewish physicians who had emigrated to other parts of Europe, and because of information sent by colonists and missionaries overseas.[15]

It is not an inconsistency or contradiction, therefore, to suggest that innovative, enlightened Portuguese *médicos* should have been trained at the pedagogically conservative University of Coimbra. Nor should we think it strange that such broad-minded physicians and surgeons should have joined the ranks of the Inquisition as mid-echelon functionaries. Other exigencies were at work at the time. Even after having been trained under outmoded Jesuit principles,

---

12   Arquivo Nacional da Torre do Tombo, Lisbon (hereafter ANTT), Inventário das habilitações do Santo Ofício, *livros* 450-471, *maço* 111, *número* 1874.

13   Maximiano Lemos, "Amigos de Ribeiro Sanches," in *Estudos de história da medicina peninsular* (Porto, 1916), 288-295.

14   ANTT, Inventário das habilitações do Santo Ofício, *livros* 450-471, *maço* 126, *número* 2227; Sousa Dias, "Equívocos," 8.

15   Maximiano Lemos, *História de medicina em Portugal: doutrinas e instituições* (Lisbon, 1991), 2: 59-154.

Coimbra graduates were still subject to exterior professional influences. Some corresponded with "foreignized" *estrangeirado* physicians; others were members of foreign learned societies; many read (often smuggled) medical publications from France, the Netherlands or Britain that advocated the effectiveness of modern medicine. All of these activities were in keeping with the heady spirit of the *Época das Luzes* (Era of Lights), of which many contemporary medical professionals – despite their archaic official training and insulated situation within Portugal – were active participants.

Men who held posts on the Coimbra faculty of medicine could hold rationalist medical principles in high esteem, though they were restricted from teaching such concepts openly within the University. Examples were numerous of Coimbra graduates, and even some *lentes de medicina* (medical instructors), who clearly favored (and often wrote about) progressive medical developments outside the official university curriculum. This was particularly true during the third quarter of the eighteenth century, as the political and cultural mood across Portugal began to display more openness under a new royal regime.[16]

All the while, many of these same enlightened physicians and surgeons simultaneously applied to become Holy Office functionaries, the valuable benefits from holding a *familiar*'s post being highly desirable and frequently sought. Further, many licensed medical practitioners who joined the Inquisition were, again in concordance with the rationalist philosophy they espoused, engaged in the persecution of illicit healers. Yet they still were bound to respect the ancient traditions of their *alma mater* and the Holy Mother Church, together with the more compelling royal laws that enforced the continuation of Coimbra's outdated curriculum.

The intellectually constrained situation within the *Faculdade de Medicina* would not change until the period between 1759 and 1772, when the prime minister, Pombal, was powerful enough to suppress the Jesuits and reorganize the universities. Only at that time was every discipline taught at Coimbra thoroughly recast and given a state-prescribed curriculum, methodology and examination standards based on modern principles.[17] In the medical field, this would entail the re-introduction of human dissection as the basis of

---

16   For notable examples, see Augusto do Silva Carvalho, *Dicionário dos médicos e cirurgiões portugueses ou que estiveram em Portugal*, unpublished typescript with manuscript annotations, 32 volumes, Biblioteca da Academia das Ciências de Lisboa (1949?), 2: 203 (Casimir de Costa Caetano); 3: 24 (António Dias Inchado); 3: 113-114 (José Ferreira da Moura); 5: 152 (Manuel Mendes de Sousa Trovão); 6: 47 (António Nunes); 8: 90 (Bernardo Silva e Moura); and 8: 170-171 (Inácio do Valle).

17   Joaquim Verríssimo Serrão, *História de Portugal*, 10 vols. (Lisbon, 1996), 4: 268.

anatomical study, as well as the adoption of more recent medical doctrines, including Harvey's teaching regarding blood circulation, Albinus' concepts in anatomy, van Sweiten's in pharmacology and Boerhaave's in pathology. The study of hygiene as a preventative health care measure would, in accordance with Pombal's wishes, also be introduced at Coimbra in 1772.[18] Before that date, however, many practicing licensed *médicos* across Portugal had already begun to follow the currents of change from abroad that managed to reach their peculiarly peripheral country.

Prior to Pombal's reforms, the knowledge of pathology and the assessment of treatments was, among the general Iberian medical community, still basically Galenic.[19] Similarly, during the middle 1700s, medical theorists in Portugal as elsewhere were only beginning to develop an understanding of the importance of sanitation and proper hygiene to good health.

How one approached treating illness was, in this era, largely socio-economically determined, and the two worlds of elite and popular medicine in Portugal, as elsewhere, rarely met on the same ground. State-licensed healers typically did not share a common cultural approach to healing with their prospective patients among the peasantry. They invariably followed the tenets of humoral medicine and mostly resorted to the lancet to draw quantities of blood. Moreover, conventional practitioners of medicine were, for rural people with access to little ready money, expensive. In the eyes of a rustic tenant farmer and his family, it must have seemed that the odds of being cured by a *curandeiro* or *saludador* were no different from those derived from any treatment a licensed surgeon or physician could provide. So, common people in Portugal had little incentive to patronize the few licensed doctors and surgeons they were likely to encounter in the countryside or provincial towns.[20]

Exacerbating the problem of poor medical training within Portugal further, medical publications from the rest of contemporary Europe were often stopped at the border. The Portuguese government tried to impede unorthodox ideas and sentiments from crossing into Portugal, using censorship as a means to keep unwanted doctrines out of the cognizance of the people. The crown

---

18   Kenneth Maxwell, *Pombal: Paradox of the Enlightenment* (Cambridge, 1995), 102; and Lemos, *História*, 2: 185-197.

19   Arturo Castiglioni, *A History of Medicine* (New York, 1975), 350-351, 700-701. See also Lemos, *História*, 2: 59-154.

20   See Charles R. Boxer, "Some Remarks on the Social and Professional Status of Physicians and Surgeons in the Iberian World, 16th-18th Centuries," *Jornal da Sociedade das Ciências médicas de Lisboa*, 137 (1974), 287-306; Maria Benedita Araújo, *O conhecimento empírico dos fármacos nos séculos XVII e XVIII* (Lisbon, 1992), 21-32; José Pedro Paiva, *Práticas e crenças mágicas na diocese de Coimbra (1650-1740)* (Coimbra, 1992), 77-119.

called on the Holy Office in the seventeenth century to help administer this effort, forming a Royal Board of Censorship (*Mesa de censura*) that empowered Inquisition employees to search ships and homes for prohibited materials. During the early stages of the Enlightenment, the Inquisition increased its vigilance, initiating trials not just against persons holding heretical religious texts, but also people of learning who dared question the (largely Jesuit-determined) educational *status quo*.

For the medical profession, the impact of this policy was to severely restrict most professional Portuguese physicians' access to the new theories and practical knowledge emanating from centers of medical learning in the Netherlands, France and Britain. Still, as Enlightenment historian José Sebastião Dias has noted, "determined thinkers ... managed to obtain and circulate [banned scientific] books."[21] A great irony, in fact, in the history of Portuguese medical modernization is that, beginning approximately in the 1720s, many of the most ardent and active advocates for reform were themselves employees of the Inquisition, who used their privileged positions to gain access to prohibited medical and scientific texts.

The Role of Licensed Medical Practitioners within the Inquisition

Trained physicians and surgeons found a comfortable place within the hierarchy of the Holy Office, where their particular skills were essential to the day-to-day functioning of Inquisition business. Their numbers within the organization were always relatively small, limited by the few official medical posts open to them, until the late seventeenth century, when employment as a *familiar* became more fashionable among ambitious men of the growing learned professional class in Portugal.[22] The earliest association of medical professionals with the Inquisition stemmed from the need to have a doctor resident in or attached officially to the Inquisition prisons. Each regional tribunal in Portugal – Lisbon, Évora and Coimbra – maintained its own facilities for the incarceration of prisoners awaiting trial or exile, or for the imprisonment of those serving sentences after being convicted of a wide variety of crimes. Prisons being notoriously unhealthy places, and the Holy Office being in some measure sensitive to its responsibility for the health of persons held under its jurisdiction, the need for approved medical personnel attached to the Inquisition *cárceres* was manifest.

---

21   Silva Dias, *Portugal*, 292-295.
22   Viega Torres, "Da repressão religiosa," 127-135.

The 1640 *Regimento* of the Portuguese Inquisition, the primary manual of regulations which governed every function of that organization until 1774 (when the *Regimento* was revised in accordance with Pombaline reforms), provided specifically for the appointment of designated dedicated professional medical staff: one doctor, one surgeon and a barber in each city where a tribunal of the Holy Office resided (though in practice inquisitors might call for medical expertise on any other licensed healers who were also *familiares*).[23] Medical officials were chosen according to the rigorous standards applied to any Inquisition employee – all physicians, surgeons and barbers who wished to work for the Inquisition first had to submit to the process of becoming a *familiar* of the Holy Office. Such a vetting process involved an intensive background check to verify that the applicant was an "Old Christian" of pure blood, untainted by that of any ancestors who had been converted to Christianity. Further, the applicant had to be of sound moral and social standing; to ascertain this, the Inquisition took depositions from friends and professional associates who vouched for the character of the applicant. Candidates endured an obligatory investigation of their sources of income, mental stability, civic virtue and moral reputation. Moreover, the wives or fiancées, parents and grandparents of would-be Inquisition functionaries had to undergo similar examinations to prove, in accordance with the "purity of blood" requirement, that their lineage was free of any New Christian taint.[24]

Working inside the Inquisition prisons, of course, implied access to and knowledge of Inquisition methods; strict secrecy always shrouded the internal functioning of the organization, and all employees were bound alike by the terms of their positions to maintain a unified front against prying outsiders.[25] *Familiares* were paid generally well, either by the day or on a fee basis for their services. Professional medical personnel, however, drew an additional salary, the amount of which was set at the time of their appointment and seems to have varied according to the personal circumstances of each appointee.[26]

From the physicians' point of view, initiating an association with the Holy Office was especially desirable for other reasons. Becoming a *familiar* brought

23 *Regimento do Santo Officio da Inquisição dos Reynos de Portugal. Ordenado por mandado do ilustrissimo e reverendissimo senhor Bispo Dom Francisco de Castro, Inquisidor Geral do Concelho de Estado de Sua Magestade* (Lisbon, 1640), *Livro* I, *Titulo* 1, § 1. See also Baudry's article in this volume.

24 Gustav Henningsen and John Tedeschi, eds., *The Inquisition in Early Modern Europe: Studies on Sources and Methods* (Dekalb, Ill., 1986), 83-84.

25 *Regimento do Santo Officio* (1640), *Livro* I, *Titulo* I, § 7. See also "Regimento dos familiares do Santo Oficio" (1694), British Library, London, MS Add. 20: 953, fols. 173-174.

26 *Regimento do Santo Officio* (1640), *Livro* II, *Titulo* XX, § 4; *Livro* II, *Titulo* XXI, § 5.

many tangible social benefits. Employees of the Inquisition were exempt from military service, general taxation, and from the requisitioning of their lodgings by the government for the use of troops or officials. *Familiares* were shown special favor in the distribution of fundamental consumer goods, such as bread, meat, fish, olive oil, wood and coal, during times of dearth or emergency. Moreover, Inquisition functionaries lived beyond the reach of royal jurisdiction; they were answerable only to the law courts of the Holy Office. This was true whether an Inquisition employee was the accused or the plaintiff in a criminal trial, or if he were a defendant in a civil lawsuit.[27] These extraordinary perquisites annoyed the common citizenry, who protested Inquisition privileges steadily over the years of the institution's activity.

Perhaps it was this popular resentment that prompted the issue of a revised *Regimento* pertaining only to *familiares* in 1694. This brief statement, printed for public distribution, further defined and restricted the rights of Inquisition civil employees with an explicit view toward minimizing friction between them and the general public. Written prominently into the opening paragraphs is a caveat for *familiares* against immodest comportment and dress that "might result in prejudice against the *Santo Ofício*." Inquisition authorities, concerned about antagonizing the general population, warned employees not to "aggravate or vex" any person by invoking Holy Office privileges, lest common citizens develop "hatred" for such behavior.[28] In particular, this publication warned that *familiares* could not receive special discounts from merchants or favors from royal officials who might have other business with the Holy Office. Beyond that, the document stipulated that *familiares* "could not accept any item, even if it be of little value" from members of the public, lest someone expect special consideration in return. For a *familiar* to do so would be to risk suspension from duty – and the consequent cessation of the privileges of office.[29]

Nevertheless, such castigation did not reduce the demand for posts within the Holy Office; indeed, the opposite was true. Among *letrados* – educated elites such as lawyers, scholars and, of course, physicians – desire to become a *familiar* grew steadily, expanding during the century from 1670 to 1770. According to a valuable study published in 1994 by José Viega Torres, the number of *familiares* employed by the Inquisition during this period grew by a factor greater than 4.5 times. During the decade from 1661 to 1670, there were a total of 478 *familiares* attached to the three tribunals of Lisbon, Évora and Coimbra; by contrast, 2252 *familiares* worked for the Holy Office during the decade 1761-

27   Henningsen and Tedeschi, *The Inquisition,* 84.
28   "Regimento dos Familiares do Santo Ofício," fols. 173-174.
29   Ibid.

1770. Using the same decades, twenty-nine of the Inquisition's 478 *familiares* were *letrados* during the earlier period; one hundred years later the number had grown to 260. In the period 1741 to 1750, the last decade of Dom João V's reign, fully 11% (182 of 1639) of *familiares* were identified professionally as *letrados*, a sizable proportion of whom were *médicos*.[30]

Torres argued convincingly that the rising middle class in Portugal grasped the utility of a *familiar*'s credentials as a way to enhance their social status and gain practical social advantages. Increasingly, he said, the Inquisition became an institution that promoted the interests of the Old Christian bourgeoisie: learned professionals, state bureaucrats and urban merchants alike. Professional medical practitioners followed this trend like so many of their social peers, seeking to increase their status, participate in the Inquisition network and gain the perquisites of office consequent to being a *familiar*.

To lend a further dimension of understanding to this matter, consider the statistically significant number of all Portuguese physicians and surgeons who worked for the Inquisition in varying capacities during the reign of Dom João V. Portuguese historian of medicine Augusto da Silva Carvalho's massive eight-volume work, *Dicionário dos Médicos e Cirurgiões Portugueses ou que estiveram em Portugal*, an unpublished typescript with manuscript annotations completed in about 1940, lists alphabetically an estimated 12,000 medical practitioners who were active in Portugal between the thirteenth and the first half of the twentieth centuries. An examination of these volumes yielded approximately 2100 listings for the period between 1690 and 1760. Of these, there were 1948 entries containing enough detailed information about the life of the named physician or surgeon to ascertain accurately whether or not he was a functionary of the Holy Office. Nearly 8% of those entries (150 of 1948) had acquired credentials as *familiares* of the Inquisition.[31] While this cannot be considered a complete listing and we must allow for a sizable margin of error, these figures are reasonably consistent with those Torres offers for the number of *letrados* who became *familiars* of the Inquisition during this period when the overall number of *familiares* was also expanding.

For a further check to give insight into this subject, a survey of the indexes for records of applications to the Holy Office, the *habilitações do Santo Ofício*, reveals that only approximately 4% of all those wishing to become *familiares* during the first half of the eighteenth century were either licensed physicians,

---

30   Viega Torres, "Da repressão religiosa," 127-133.
31   Silva Carvalho, *Dicionário dos Médicos*, volumes 1-8.

surgeons, barbers, phlebotomists or pharmacists. However, the great majority of these – better than 95% – were ultimately approved for service.[32]

Since this essay was first published in 2007, further archival research into these records has revealed additional information. A comprehensive survey of the *habilitações do Santo Ofício* collection, conducted by the author between 2008 and 2011, turned up abundant further evidence of active participation by licensed physicians and surgeons (as well as a few barbers and phlebotomists) in the ranks of the Portuguese Inquisition. This survey uncovered a total of 245 medical professions from across Portugal who applied for and were granted the credentials to become *familiars* of the Holy Office in Portugal between 1690 and 1778.[33] And why not? Medical practitioners, because of their peculiar professional activities, made excellent agents for the Holy Office. As *familiars*, they were respected, learned members of society and often had access to dimensions of their patients' lives that normally would be veiled to outsiders.

Two further examples from the survey demonstrate how influential and closely linked the professional lives of these physicians could be to the Inquisition, the Royal Court, and the University of Coimbra. On 22 August 1707, António Simões da Silva was granted his *carta de familiar* (Holy Office credentials) as a member of the Coimbra tribunal. Da Silva, born in the influential Coimbra *freguesia* of São Pedro, had earned a doctorate in Coimbra and risen to become a professor of medicine there. He served the crown as well, as a designated physician of the Royal Household (*Médico de Real Câmara*).[34] The Holy Office approved da Silva's application shortly after young King João v ascended the throne; the leadership of the Inquisition changed that year, too, when the new king nominated Coimbra native Dom Nuno da Cunha de Ataíde e Mello as Inquisitor General.[35] Two years later, da Silva's younger colleague, physician João Pessoa da Fonseca, also an instructor in the faculty of medicine at the University of Coimbra, received his *carta de familiar* on 14 November 1709. Fonseca had been born in the prosperous neighborhood of Coimbra, as well.[36]

By using the rich demographic detail found in the individual application dossiers (*habilitações*) of the Holy Office, combined with Inquisition trial records, a vivid personal portrait of licensed Portuguese practitioners of medicine in the early modern period can emerge. The survey provides a broad social assessment of the persons who entered the medical profession in early mod-

---

32   ANTT, Inventário das habilitações do Santo Ofício, *livros* 450-471, vols. 1-32.

33   Ibid.

34   ANTT, Inventário das habilitações do Santo Ofício, *livros* 450-471, *maço* 49, *número* 1084.

35   Maria Luísa Braga, *A Inquisição em Portugal, primeira metade do séc. XVIII: o Inquisidor Geral D. Nuno da Cunha de Athayde e Mello* (Lisbon, 1992), 25-32.

36   ANTT, Inventário das habilitações do Santo Ofício, *livros* 450-471, *maço* 45, *número* 908.

ern Portugal. Such documentation can help to explain how, during the period in question, entering the medical profession was one means by which literate men (*letrados*) from modest families could improve their social status and, through joining the Inquisition, influence national policies toward medicine and healing.

Simultaneously, the survey helps to demonstrate how physicians and surgeons in the late seventeenth and eighteenth centuries became part of a growing professional middle class (barbers and bloodletters, by contrast, though required to be licensed, did not share the same social or professional standing as their more learned colleagues). Because of their enhanced status as university-trained, state-licensed healers – the only social group officially recognized and sanctioned to care for human illness – *médicos* and *cirurgiões* became more aware of themselves as a distinct professional and social group. Adding to this dynamic, contemporary Portuguese elites increasingly began to demand that royal government authorities credential conventional healers. The faculty of medicine at the University of Coimbra, the royal *Todos-os-Santos* hospital in Lisbon, and the tribunals of the Inquisition became nodes of association for medical professionals. These institutions provided an environment where licensed practitioners of medicine became more conscious of the need to professionalize, as well as to the benefits of increased professionalization. Licensed medical practitioners began to guard the parameters of their profession more closely, becoming more protective of healing standards and licensing criteria. As I have indicated, this dynamic is reflected in the spate of contemporary Inquisition magical crimes trials conducted against popular folk healers during the eighteenth century.

To underscore the enhanced influence that affiliation with the Holy Office could bring to a licensed medical practitioner, consider the early case of prominent Lisbon surgeon António Ferreira, who from the 1660s served in the royal chamber of King Pedro II, and in 1662 accompanied princess Catarina of Bragança to London for her marriage to King Charles II. For more than twenty years he was a surgeon of Lisbon's *Todos-os-Santos* hospital. In 1670 Ferreira published what would become a highly regarded and successful book on surgery, entitled *Luz verdadyra e recopilado exame de toda a cirurgia*; by 1757 this work had gone through four editions.[37] On the title page of the 1683 and 1705 editions, António Ferreira's achievements and affiliations were proudly

37   Laurinda Abreu, "A organização e regulação das *profissões médicas* no Portugal moderno: entre as orientações da coroa e os interesses privados," in Adelino Cardoso, António Braz de Oliveira, Manuel Silvério Marques, eds., *Arte médica e imagem do corpo: ee Hipócrates ao final do séc. XVIII* (Lisbon, 2010), 107-122; and her *Public Health and Social Reforms in Portugal (1780-1805)* (Cambridge, 2017), 210-11.

proclaimed: besides being named surgeon to the king's chambers, he was a "surgeon of the prisons of the Holy Office, and familiar of that institution, and of the *Tribunal da relação* of the Royal Court [a crown judiciary body that heard appeals cases], and a professed Knight of the Order of Our Lord Jesus Christ."[38] Clearly, here was a man of exceptional influence, whose social and political connections linked him to the top policy makers in the country. Ferreira's circumstances are noteworthy but far from unique, historically, among conspicuous medical men in Portugal who served the Crown and Inquisition.

The Inquisition quite naturally sought to fill its ranks with the best possible candidates, men of unquestioned reputation and moral standing, but also of notable skill in their work. Indeed, the 1640 *Regimento* stipulated that Inquisition medical staff should be persons "worthy of great confidence," and the "best informed individuals of the town."[39] And of course, because of the benefits derived from Holy Office employment, the best eligible Old Christian medical practitioners sought positions there to further enhance their own social status. In fact, as José Viega Torres suggests, the Inquisition functioned increasingly during the eighteenth century as something of a fraternal trade organization where members "networked," developing social and professional contacts, and reinforced thereby their position in the community.[40]

Membership usually brought increased status, true, but facilitated real material benefit, as well. It should come as no surprise, then, that the Holy Office drew to its ranks some of the best-known physicians and surgeons of the day, and that, because of their renown, these were often exactly the same men who were tapped to fill posts both at the royal court and at hospitals and the university (Coimbra) supported by the crown. Plurality of office was, as elsewhere in Europe, quite common in eighteenth-century Portugal, and the number of qualified physicians and surgeons was always relatively small.

It is for this reason that a modestly-sized interconnected group of elite medical professionals could come to exercise a significant influence over several key Portuguese institutions just before and during the reign of João v; many of the same surgeons and physicians simultaneously held posts in the Inquisition, at court, in the royal *Todos-os-Santos* hospital in Lisbon (important as a teaching hospital), and in the faculty of medicine of the University of Coimbra. Moreover, because such posts were often lifetime appointments, these men held their positions typically for decades at a time, throughout the most

---

38   António Ferreira, *Luz verdadeyra, e recopilado exame de toda a cirurgia* (Lisbon, 1683); 1705
        edition published in Lisbon.
39   *Regimento do Santo Officio* (1640), *Livro* I, *Titulo* XX, § 1.
40   Viega Torres, "Da repressão religiosa," 122-123; 131-132.

important, productive years of their careers. Hence, this central corps of medical professionals exercised an influence at the core of the Portuguese *ancien regime* that was marked by great consistency and continuity. Many of the key faces stayed the same for much of João V's reign.

Once approved, an Inquisition *médico* could expect to carry out a variety of duties. Significantly, in addition to the inmates of the Inquisition prisons, the physician and surgeon of the three regional Holy Office tribunals were obliged by the terms of their appointment to care for the officers of those tribunals, as well as for members of these inquisitors' respective families. It was for this reason that the Inquisition supplied a salary to its medical employees, according to the 1640 *Regimento*.[41] Thus, the administrative personnel of the Holy Office were provided with their own in-house health care service, staffed by the most esteemed licensed professionals of the realm.

The working interaction between these two classes of Inquisition employees should have been wholly amicable. This was, after all, a relationship between peers; both physicians and upper-level inquisitors were social elites of similar upbringing who enjoyed a great deal of status due to their positions as part of a small class of educated professionals, as well as for their association with the Holy Office. These men were, generally speaking, drawn from a similar stratum of society and shared kindred background experiences: Old Christian families, usually of equitable economic means; long association with the church; similar educational training; possible patronage from a noble or aristocratic family; and a particular consciousness born of belonging to an elevated social class in relation to most other people in early modern Portuguese society.

What principal duties occupied the time of a physician or surgeon assigned to oversee an Inquisition prison? Squalid, ill lit and poorly ventilated, the *cárceres* of the Holy Office, like any early modern prison, provided a propitious environment for disease.[42] Because accused persons often remained incarcerated for months and even years, many inmates succumbed to illness. The *médico dos cárceres*, along with the surgeon and barber, were charged with maintaining, to the best of their abilities, good health among the prisoners. Toward this end, they were required to make regular rounds, bleeding inmates

---

41   *Regimento do Santo Officio* (1640), *Livro* I, *Titulo* XX, § 3.

42   Those interested in the state of Inquisition prisons can still read accounts published in English by merchants arrested for freemasonry, such as John Coustos, *The Sufferings of John Coustos for Free Masonry and for Refusing to turn Roman Catholic in the Inquisition at Lisbon...* (London, 1746) and Hippolyto Joseph da Costa Pereira Furtado de Mendonça, *Narrative of the Persecution of Hyppolyto Joseph da Costa Pereira Furtado de Mendonça...*, 2 vols. (London, 1811), 1: 138-139.

whose humors were clearly out of balance, prescribing changes in diet, and dispensing medicinal preparations, usually at the prisoner's expense.[43]

Beyond treating inmates for the inevitable maladies which arose from their unfavorable living conditions, Inquisition physicians and surgeons examined prisoners to see if they were fit enough physically and mentally to undergo torture sessions. That the prisoner be able to endure prolonged pain and remain conscious to give testimony was essential to the interrogation process. If the physician or surgeon judged the prisoner to be of a sound constitution, that medical practitioner would also attend the torture session to supply a professional opinion about the state of the prisoner as the session progressed. The physician or surgeon could determine if the treatment should proceed, or whether torture had begun to endanger the life of the accused.[44] Inquisition records clearly show many cases where torture sessions were halted because, in the attending medical practitioner's view, the victim's threshold of pain had been passed, after which point the prisoner ceased to be a valuable witness.[45]

Occasionally the *médico dos cárceres* would be summoned to attend an especially grave case, either at the request of the chief jailer or of the prisoner's family. And occasionally this system of responsibility broke down. For example, in Coimbra in 1741, Clara Maria da Costa, aged twenty-six, was arrested for suspicion of perpetrating superstitious acts and sorcery. Re-arrested for a relapse of her objectionable ways eleven years later, she fell gravely ill while in the regional Bishop's prison at Oporto. The latter third of her official Inquisition dossier is full of letters, written by family members or friends and dated from the late 1750s, petitioning for her release on the grounds that she was both innocent and in poor health. Although the physician of the Royal Arsenal at Oporto examined her and certified that she was gravely ill, the *alcaide* (jailer) in charge of the prison would not release her without the consent of surgeon Manuel Martims Freire, who was the official *médico dos cárceres* in Coimbra and a *familiar* of the Inquisition. For some unspecified reason, probably because of the distances and time involved, Freire never travelled to Oporto to examine the accused prisoner. As late as 1771, Clara Maria da Costa remained incarcerated, appealing her case.[46] In that year she was approximately fifty-six years old and had spent better than twenty years in prison.

If a convict or one of the accused became mentally unstable while incarcerated, the chief jailer and inquisitors would call upon the prison medical staff to

---

43   *Regimento do Santo Officio* (1640), *Livro* I, *Titulo* XX, § 2-4.

44   Ibid., § 6.

45   ANTT, Inquisição de Coimbra, *processos* nos. 9545 and 7346; Inquisiçao de Évora, *processos* nos. 516 and 2602.

46   ANTT, Inquisição de Coimbra, *processo* no. 6299.

address the prisoner's madness. Judging from the explicitness with which "insanity" was addressed in the 1640 *Regimento*, this problem, whether feigned or real, was not uncommon. And no wonder: then as now, being judged mentally deficient worked to the accused's advantage. Legal proceedings against the suspect were suspended and the prison physicians were ordered to restore the inmate to his senses with "all possible means," including whatever medicines they thought necessary. If in the physicians' opinion the prescribed remedy could not be administered effectively within the *cárceres*, the prisoner would be interned at the *Todos-os-Santos* hospital in Lisbon, which had a special ward to treat madness. The 1640 *Regimento* further provided that, should the accused patient still not regain his or her senses, they would be released to the care of his relatives until such time as they were judged able to stand trial, if at all.[47]

Periodically doctors of the Inquisition would be called to testify during a trial, where they were expected to give a professional opinion in cases against popular healers or sorcerers. In a sworn statement, the physician would provide an opinion about why, from the viewpoint of scientific medicine, the accused was a charlatan. Statements such as these range from the perfunctory to ones of exceptional detail, with the *médico* giving a lengthy explanation of why a *curandeiro's* methods were unsound. For example, in 1714, when doctor Gonçalves de Ferreira testified against the accused healer Maria Álvares, he described specifically the maladies for which she had been consulted and saying with all the weight of his medical authority that her treatments were ill matched to the symptoms her patients displayed.[48] Or consider another case, this one against a male healer named Paulo Simões, in 1700. After an initial statement given by one Manuel Luís, a merchant of Coimbra, accusing Paulo Simões of being in the habit of performing cures with blessings (*costuma curar com bençōes*), there follows a statement from Doctor António Teixeira Álvares, surgeon and "doctor of the Algarve, instructor of the University of Coimbra and *Promotor* [prosecutor] of the city." He essentially confirmed and supported the case against the accused by reiterating the charges, his very presence affirming that the healer's methods were medically unsound.[49]

Inquisition doctors and surgeons were also instrumental in the mandatory investigations that followed the death of any prisoner held in the Holy Office prisons. The 1640 *Regimento* governing the Inquisition required that the remains of a deceased prisoner be examined "before the body is removed from

---

47   *Regimento do Santo Officio* (1640), *Livro* II, *Titulo* XVII, § 1-2.

48   ANTT, Inquisição de Coimbra, *processo* no. 8698.

49   ANTT, Inquisição de Coimbra, *processo* no. 9711.

the room wherein he died" by "two notaries and one of the physicians of the Holy Office" so that these officials could ascertain whether the death had been the result of violence or natural causes (murder and suicide among inmates of Inquisition prisons was apparently not unknown).[50] For example, during the second quarter of the eighteenth century, the physician Manuel dos Reis e Sousa was called upon several times during his tenure as *médico* of the Inquisition prisons in Coimbra to certify the cause of death when a prisoner expired while in custody. In a signed *Acto do Morte*, the doctor affirmed that the prisoner had succumbed to natural causes and was not the victim of undue ill treatment or foul play.[51]

An Inquisition physician might also have been called in to examine a prisoner for medical evidence of being a crypto-Jew. Diogo Nunes Brandão, a New Christian born in Lisbon in 1671, had trained in medicine at the University of Coimbra. He was arrested on 3 August 1702 by the Inquisition of Lisbon and charged with *judaismo*. As part of the initial investigation into his case, Inquisition authorities arranged to have him undergo a physical examination conducted by the *médico* Manuel de Pina Coutinho and a surgeon, António de Figueiredo, both *familiares* of the Holy Office. The two medical practitioners, apparently called in to give a second opinion on an earlier examination, declared that a scar which the accused had next to what they termed his "gland" was the result of horseback riding and specifically not the mark of a circumcision. Despite this evidence in his favor, Brandão confessed to all his beliefs and practices as a Jew and proceeded to denounce more than one hundred of his co-religionists in both Portugal and Spain. He was condemned to perform penances and serve an indefinite imprisonment at the discretion of the inquisitors on 3 October 1704.[52]

Clearly, physicians and surgeons were central to the internal bureaucracy of the Holy Office. In addition to attending to the health of incarcerated offenders, they also participated in each stage of a *processo* from beginning to end: examining the accused person during an initial investigation, providing testimony as expert witnesses, overseeing torture sessions and, in cases against popular healers, submitting professional statements assessing the efficacy of the accused's healing practices.

Because they also tended to the illnesses of the inquisitors themselves and their families, and because these learned professionals interacted frequently

---

50   *Regimento do Santo Officio* (1640), *Livro* II, *Titulo* XVIII, § 1.

51   ANTT, Inquisição de Coimbra, *processos* nos. 7300, 6315 and 6218.

52   ANTT, Inquisição de Lisboa, *processos* nos. 15292 and 2361; see also Silva Carvalho, *Dicionário dos Médicos*, 6: 72-73.

on a social plane that was more or less level, physicians and surgeons were uniquely placed to influence Holy Office policies regarding popular healers. After all, it was the *médicos*, their families or subordinate colleagues – *sangradors* and *barbeiros* – who initiated many of the trials against *curandeiros* by denouncing them to the Holy Office. The immediate effect of the Inquisition's persecution of *curandeiros* during this period was to serve the interests of professional medical practitioners.

The Inquisitors' Point of View

Persecuting healers also served the interests of the inquisitors who directed the Holy Office. However, interests at the top of the institution were substantially different from those of contemporary doctors within the lower ranks of the Inquisition. By bringing popular healers to trial, high ranking inquisitors hoped to assert and perpetuate the role of their institution within Portuguese society. Naturally, the Inquisition's mission was to confront heresy or apostasy in any of its manifestations, and to compel orthodox behavior among Catholics living in regions under its jurisdiction. Therefore, to pursue cases of superstitious healers who, in the eyes of the church, relied on nefarious ungodly powers for their efficacy was clearly consistent with the original purpose of the Inquisition.

Further, such ecclesiastical policing justified the continued existence of the Inquisition at a critical moment when that institution was being criticized by persons inside and outside of Portugal who charged that the Holy Office, an anachronistic, reactionary body, was retarding Portugal's progress among the other nations of a modernizing Europe. The propaganda war against the Inquisition, conducted by *estrangeirado* expatriates and Protestants from northern Europe, was at full tide during the middle years of the eighteenth century.[53] A prolonged campaign against supposed agents of Satan (and, not incidentally, against Jews, who also found themselves more vigorously persecuted during this period)[54] demonstrated that the need for continued vigilance in the face of demonic activity had not abated. Finally, a strong stance against the spiritual enemies of the Catholic Church reinforced the Inquisition's reputation

---

53   See the writings of António Nunes Ribeiro Sanches, among other key works, *Origem da denominação de cristão-velho e cristão-novo em Portugal* (1756), as well as Coustos, *The Sufferings* (1746).

54   Walker, *Doctors*, 50-54; 89-90; 103; 119-132.

and position in the popular mind as protectors of the faith, guarantors of the common people's salvation.

For the majority of the Portuguese people, persecutions of Jews and heretics remained a popularly supported crusade; therefore, such trials, even if they drew criticism from intellectuals abroad, represented a net public relations victory for the Inquisition.[55] Still, we must remember: in the case of *curandeiros*, these benefits accrued to the Holy Office only as a secondary effect of the doctor/*familiares'* initial actions. Left to themselves, Inquisition and church officials in the seventeenth century had taken almost no interest in or action against folk healers. Systematic persecution of *curandeiros* required a critical mass of licensed medical professionals engaged in the ranks of the Portuguese Holy Office.

Hence, we have an extraordinary situation in which two bodies of individuals within the same institution – the *médicos* and the inquisitors – were working toward widely divergent ends by pursuing the same course of action. By bringing popular healers to trial and charging them with crimes against God – superstition, sorcery and witchcraft – medical professionals sought to reinforce their own position, both economically and authoritatively, within the medical field. Moreover, by discrediting popular healers, progressive-minded doctors simultaneously sought to further the cause of rational scientific medicine within Portugal. The inquisitors, conversely, attempted to reinforce their position as guardians of the faith by insisting on the maintenance of a *status quo* in medicine which had existed in Portugal for four hundred years: the subordination of medical training under a framework consistent with Church orthodoxy, as characterized by Galenic teaching. This view included the continuance of the position that assumed that all popular healers necessarily derived illicit powers from diabolical sources, a view which more than justified their persecution. The Holy Office had nothing to gain by introducing the population at large to medical innovations; on the contrary, the church had a long record of resisting scientific discoveries that contradicted orthodox teaching precisely because science undermined the church's institutional authority.

Even so, as the Inquisition recognized implicitly by employing *médicos* as *familiares*, trained doctors could be very useful in ferreting out dangerous *curandeiros*. It was a most contradictory relationship. Folk healers, for their part, were caught in the middle: not only were they undermining the professional authority of scientifically trained doctors; they were also challenging the church's spiritual authority either implicitly or explicitly by claiming powers of

---

55   Francisco Bethencourt, *História das Inquisições: Portugal, Espanha e Itália* (Lisbon, 1994) 230-248.

healing which, under orthodox thought, should rightly come only from God. In so doing, *curandeiros* became targets for persecution from both groups. Inquisitors and *médicos* therefore combined against popular healers, each for their own reasons. Although science and religion embarked on increasingly divergent paths as the Enlightenment wore on, for that moment in Portugal, agents of both camps could still work together before separating, with doctors removing healing from the spiritual realm and placing it firmly into the scientific sphere.

That Portuguese Old Christian doctors had previously used the Inquisition to attack their professional competitors has already been demonstrated, though the cases they initially brought were typically against New Christian medical practitioners, not popular healers. Maria Benedita Araújo, in her article entitled *Médicos e Seus Familiares na Inquisição de Évora*, refers exclusively to New Christians and their relatives who were persecuted within the jurisdiction of the Évora tribunal of the Inquisition – the Algarve and Alentejo regions – during the sixteenth, seventeenth and eighteenth centuries.[56] She reports that, in many cases, Old Christian doctors went to officials of the Holy Office and denounced New Christian physicians and surgeons as crypto-Jews, often when the latter were young and just starting out in the medical profession.[57] Her findings reveal a pattern of persecution, too, but at a time when there were far fewer *médicos* at work in the Holy Office ranks. Nevertheless, this practice constituted a powerful precedent for Old Christian doctors, demonstrating a way that Inquisition regulations could be put to use for their own purposes. This phenomenon was also known within the jurisdiction of the Coimbra Holy Office tribunal. Knowledge of these cases helps to explain why scores of New Christian *médicos* left Portugal during the seventeenth and eighteenth centuries to take up residence abroad, becoming thereby the very *estrangeirados* who through their correspondence would so strongly influence thought about medical reform in their home country.[58]

A brief look at the working relationship between one veteran inquisitor, António Ribeiro de Abreu, who as a Holy Office prosecutor (*deputado*) conducted dozens of *curandeiro* trials in Coimbra and Lisbon, and António de Abreu Bacellar, a licensed physician who held the credentials of an Inquisition *familiar*, will provide a good picture of how close the relationship between these two types of elite professionals could be.

---

56   Maria Benedita Araújo, "Médicos e seus familiares na Inquisição de Évora," in *Comunicações apresentadas ao 1º Congresso Luso-Brasileiro Sobre Inquisição*, 3 vols. (Lisbon, 1990), 1: 49-72.

57   Ibid., 65.

58   Carneiro, et al., "The Scientific Revolution," 591-604; Walker, *Doctors,* 192-207.

António Ribeiro de Abreu and António de Abreu Bacellar worked side-by-side in Coimbra between approximately 1718 and 1730, during the middle phase of the Inquisition's long sustained period of trials against *curandeiros*. António Ribeiro de Abreu was one of the Coimbra tribunal's most active inquisitors in cases against popular healers, serving as a judge in more trials – at least twenty-four – than any other inquisitor except his contemporary, Bento Paes de Amaral.[59] António de Abreu Bacellar, meanwhile, had earned a doctorate, was a professor on the Coimbra faculty of medicine, had been a *familiar* of the Holy Office since 1699 and, beginning on 15 March 1707, was an official prison physician of the Coimbra Inquisition (*físico dos cárceres da Inquisição*).[60] He held this post into the 1730s, through the period of António Ribeiro de Abreu's tenure as an inquisitor in Coimbra. Moreover, as an indication of his philosophical outlook, António de Abreu Bacellar was personally acquainted with the progressive expatriate physician Jacob de Castro Sarmento, who advocated for rationalist medical reform in Portugal. Abreu Bacellar would correspond with the famous Portuguese *converso* Castro Sarmento, once the latter became a fugitive expatriate living and practicing medicine in London.[61]

One product of António Ribeiro de Abreu and António de Abreu Bacellar's long collaboration as functionaries of the Inquisition was a string of Holy Office trials that, taken together, amount to a campaign of persecution against popular healers. The two were more than contemporaries; they were old colleagues. They had lived and worked together at the University of Coimbra for most if not all of the first decade of the eighteenth century. António Ribeiro de Abreu earned a doctorate in canon law and was named to several high administrative posts at the university, including *vice-conservador* (vice-provost or vice-rector).[62] During the same time, António de Abreu Bacellar was serving as a professor of surgery at the university, and in 1702 he also undertook the duties of an alderman (*vereador*) for the city of Coimbra.[63] António Ribeiro de Abreu was confirmed as a *familiar* of the Inquisition in 1712. Shortly afterward he was posted to the Lisbon tribunal as a prosecutor and deputy; he returned to

---

59   Inquisitor António Ribeiro de Abreu participated as a judge in at least twenty trials conducted by the Coimbra tribunal against sixteen different accused popular healers, four of whom were tried twice, between 1718 and 1736. See ANTT, Inquisição de Coimbra, *processos* nos. 33; 6305; 6315; 6515; 7135; 7136; 7300; 7346; 7779; 7827; 8307; 8699; 8899; 9545; and 10011.

60   ANTT, Inventário das habilitações do Santo Ofício, *livros* 450-471, *maço* 33, *número* 838; and Silva Carvalho, *Dicionário dos Médicos*, 1: 26.

61   Silva Carvalho, *Dicionário dos Médicos*, 1: 26.

62   Maria do Carmo Jasmins Dias Farinha, "Ministros do Conselho geral do Santo Ofício," *Memória, Revista anual do Arquivo Nacional da Torre do Tombo*, 1 (1989), 101-163.

63   ANTT, Inventário das habilitações do Santo Ofício, *livros* 450-471, *maço* 33, *número* 838; Silva Carvalho, *Dicionário dos Médicos*, 1: 26.

Coimbra as an inquisitor in 1718.[64] António de Abreu Bacellar's career with the Holy Office had begun sooner; he was made a *familiar* of the Holy Office on 2 March 1699.[65] The two then worked within the Coimbra tribunal simultaneously between 1718 and 1731, years of very heavy *curandeiro* prosecutions. So, these two men shared some very close ties, but there is one further connection. In all probability, the two shared a common family link; strong evidence suggests that António Ribeiro de Abreu and António de Abreu Bacellar were cousins, thus providing an additional context for their cooperative working relationship.[66]

Hence, the lives of António Ribeiro de Abreu and António de Abreu Bacellar were tightly interwoven and their working relationship was important for explaining the causality of *curandeiro* trials in Portugal, but their experience was far from unique. Medical professionals and career inquisitors frequently worked together in tight-knit institutions like the Holy Office or the University of Coimbra. As members of a middle-class educated urban elite, a group of decidedly modest size, such was simply their common experience; the institutions that trained them were small and the administrative positions open to them were relatively few. Is it any wonder, then, that these two contemporaries (and others like them) should have worked together in the Holy Office toward the same end – bringing *curandeiros* to trial (though, to be sure, probably for divergent reasons)? Because of the existence of numerous inter-linking relationships like theirs, the human and professional connections necessary to make the suppression of popular medicine possible came to be firmly in place within the institutional structure of the Portuguese Holy Office.

As has been demonstrated, some Inquisition personnel functioned as experts in the prosecution of popular healer cases. Time and again, Holy Office records provide the same names of individuals who advised the panels of inquisitors that adjudicated *curandeiro* cases. A tally correlating the names of known *deputados* with Holy Office trials pursued against known popular healers reveals that just a handful of men sat in judgment on the great majority of these cases between 1715 and 1760. As in so many other episodes of Portuguese history, the key players in the arena of conflict that pitted doctors and inquisitors against folk healers were part of a rarefied, inter-connected cadre.

---

64   Farinha, "Ministros," 136.

65   ANTT, Inventário das habilitações do Santo Ofício, *livros* 450-471, *maço* 33, *número* 838; Silva Carvalho, *Dicionário dos Médicos*, 1: 26.

66   Their exact relationship is difficult to ascertain. Available sources point to their being distant cousins. See Farinha, "Ministros," 136; and ANTT, Inventário das habilitações do Santo Ofício, *livros* 450-471, *maço* 33, *número* 838.

Overseas Colonies: Medical Professionals and the Inquisition in Brazil and India

Regarding instances of medical practitioners collaborating with the Inquisition in Portuguese overseas dominions, the analysis presented here must necessarily be somewhat speculative and inconclusive. The Portuguese Inquisition tribunal that sat in Lisbon had jurisdiction over the area surrounding the imperial capital city and a strip of central Portugal, but its members also dealt with any denunciations or cases that arose in Brazil, west Africa and the Atlantic island holdings (the archipelagos of the Azores, Madeira, Cape Verdes, and São Tomé and Príncipe). Another tribunal based in Goa, India, theoretically covered the entire eastern maritime empire, the *Estado da Índia*, stretching from Mozambique to Macau.[67]

The Lisbon tribunal maintained a network of *familiares* in each of the Atlantic colonies, and also sent Holy Office functionaries on periodic judicial circuits, or "visitations," to monitor the spiritual life of the overseas enclaves.[68] Among them were almost certainly a representative handful of licensed surgeons, physicians, and phlebotomists, who served simultaneously as crown-approved colonial medical practitioners. Cadres of Inquisition *familiares* expanded markedly in the eighteenth century – Brazil had the largest group by far, dispersed throughout the colony. Persons accused of spiritual crimes in the Atlantic enclaves were first investigated by Holy Office *familiares*; if a case was found to have merit, the accused was arrested and shipped to Lisbon to undergo interrogation and stand trial.[69]

For Asia, the few surviving Goa Inquisition tribunal records do not support a systematic inquiry about associated medical professionals working with the Portuguese Holy Office tribunal in India. That said, the Goa tribunal, which functioned in India from 1560 to 1812, was over time the most active of the four established Portuguese Holy Office districts, conducting some 20,000 trials during its tenure, mainly against lapsed lower-caste Hindus who had been forcibly converted to Roman Catholicism.[70]

---

67   Bethencourt, *História*, 45-46; Bruno Feitler, "A delegacao de poderes inquisitoriais: o exemplo de Goa atraves da documentacao da Biblioteca Nacional do Rio de Janeiro," *Tempo – Revista do Departamento de Historia da Universidade Federal Fluminense*, 12 (2008), 127-148; José Pedro Paiva, "The Inquisition Tribunal in Goa: Why and for What Purpose?," *Journal of Early Modern History*, 21 (2017), 565-593.

68   Paiva, *Bruxaria*, 197-199; Bethencourt, *História*, 45-54, 168-73.

69   Paulo Drumond Braga, *A Inquisição nos Açores* (Ponta Delgada, 1997), 73-80; Bethencourt, *História*, 128-9; Viega Torres, "Da repressão religiosa," 127-135.

70   Charles Amiel and Anne Lima, *L'Inquisition de Goa: la relation de Charles Dellon (1687)* (Paris, 1997), 63-74; Maria de Jesus dos Mártires Lopes, "A Inquisição de Goa na primeira

Because the Goa tribunal was constituted and functioned in much the same way as its counterparts in continental Portugal, it had the same need for *familiares* drawn from the elite professional class of Portuguese colonists, as well as physicians and surgeons to oversee interrogation sessions that employed torture, or attend to accused persons incarcerated at the Inquisition prison in the colonial capital. There were, however, chronically few licensed Portuguese medical professionals to be found in the Indian or South American colonies on which the Holy Office could draw for these services.[71]

Even with the dearth of trained European medical personnel, the Inquisition in Goa was notoriously hostile to Portuguese physicians and surgeons who were of Jewish descent. In Goa in 1563, the *converso* physician Garcia de Orta, who served as chief physician (*físico-môr*) of the entire Portuguese eastern empire, published his seminal work on medicines from India, entitled *Coloquios dos simples e drogas e cousas medicianais da Índia*, an enormously influential book that introduced European natural philosophy to many Asian healing plants and methods.[72] But as a "New Christian" who still practiced Judaism secretly, de Orta had left Lisbon in 1534 to avoid potential Inquisition persecution. His position as a key colonial official in Goa protected him when the Inquisition tribunal commenced operations there, but after his death in 1568 he was tried and condemned as a heretic; his body was exhumed and his remains burned in an *auto-de-fé*. Few copies of his medical book, deemed a heretical text, survived subsequent efforts by the Inquisition in Goa to seek out and destroy them.[73]

For Brazil and the other Atlantic colonies, there are some few documented physicians and surgeons who had acquired credentials as Inquisition familiars when they circulated in the overseas empire, but relatively little concrete information is known about their activities.[74] The above-mentioned survey of Holy Office *habilitações* turned up fifteen separate cases of physicians or surgeons who held credentials as *familiars* of the Inquisition while practicing medicine in Brazil. Chronologically, most of these credentials were granted in the mid-

metade de Setecentos," *Mare Liberum*, 15 (1998), 107-136; Paiva, "The Inquisition Tribunal in Goa," 566-574.

71   Timothy Walker, "Acquisition and Circulation of Medical Knowledge within the Portuguese Colonial Empire during the Early Modern Period," in Daniela Bleichmar et al., eds., *Science in the Spanish and Portuguese Empires* (Stanford, 2009), 247-270.

72   Garcia de Orta, *Colóquios dos simples e drogas he cousas medicinais da Índia* (Goa, 1563); Palmira Fontes da Costa, ed., *Medicine, Trade and Empire: Garcia de Orta's Colloquies on the Simples and Drugs of India in Context* (Aldershot, 2015).

73   Jon Arrizabalaga, "Garcia de Orta in the Context of the Sephardic Diaspora," in Fontes da Costa, ed., *Medicine,* 11-32.

74   Daniela Buono Calainho, *Agentes da Fé: Familiares da Inquisição portuguesa no Brasil colonial* (São Paulo, 2006), 69-109.

eighteenth century, clustered from the 1740s to the 1760s. Geographically they tended to be, unsurprisingly, residents in the larger communities that were the economic drivers of the colony: Salvador de Bahia, Pernambuco, Ouro Preto, Rio de Janeiro.

Two of the earliest cases, from the late seventeenth century, provide representative examples of the Inquisition's agents in Brazil. On 21 March 1694, when he was granted documents confirming his status as a *familiar* of the Holy Office, Carlos Antunes de Matos was a surgeon and businessman living in Salvador de Bahia, the colonial capital. He was 33 years old, having moved to Brazil from Lisbon, his birthplace.[75] His more senior colleague, Belchior Lopes de Azevedo, received his credentials as a *familiar* on 14 November 1695. Born in northern Portugal at Viana do Castelo, a port in the Minho district, he served as the *cirurgião môr* (chief surgeon) of Pernambuco.[76] Such men were charged with maintaining vigilance over colonial communities that, from the perspective of the metropole, were widely considered to be dangerously susceptible to moral and spiritual decadence.

For the Inquisition's activities in the Atlantic island colonies, some interesting new scholarship by Brazilian and Portuguese historians has begun to explore this subject in more detail, building on Paulo Drumond Braga's groundbreaking book, *A Inquisição nos Açores* (1997).[77] To cite just one example, Brazilian scholar Aldair Carlos Rodrigues recounted how, in 1776, Antônio Roiz Pereira, a licensed physician trained at Coimbra and an active *familiare* of the Inquisition living in Funchal, Madeira, wrote to the Holy Office in Lisbon to denounce a group of prominent persons whom he believed were guilty of secretly practicing *judaismo*. This initiated a series of trials that for years disrupted social life in that small insular community, perhaps not coincidentally just at the time that the madeira wine trade was reaching a peak in economic importance to the island, with exports throughout the Atlantic world.[78]

• • •

---

75   ANTT, Inventário das habilitações do Santo Ofício, *livros* 450-471, *maço* 1, *número* 5.
76   ANTT, Inventário das habilitações do Santo Ofício, *livros* 450-471, *maço* 3, *número* 40.
77   Braga, *A Inquisição nos Açores*; see also Flavio Coelho Edler, "Saber médico e poder profissional: do contexto luso-brasileiro ao Brasil imperial," in Carlos Fideles Ponte and Ialê Falleiros, eds., *Na corda bamba de sombrinha: a saúde no fio da história* (Rio de Janeiro, 2010), 25-46; Vinicius Cranek Gagliardo, "Condições de saúde no Brasil Colônia: primórdios da higiene pública como política governamental no Rio de Janeiro dos vice-reis," *Brasiliana. Journal for Brazilian Studies*, 2 (2013), 450-476.
78   Aldair Carlos Rodrigues, "Sociedade e Inquisição em Minas colonial: os familiars do Santo Ofício (1711-1808)" (MA thesis, Universidade de São Paulo, 2007), 113; David Hancock, *Oceans of Wine: Madeira and the Emergence of American Trade and Taste* (New Haven, 2009), 107-132.

The increase of medical professionals among the *familiar's* ranks accounts most for the dramatic growth in Inquisition cases against *saludadors* and *curandeiros* in Portugal during the reign of João V. Such medical professionals had a twofold interest in seeing popular healers oppressed and their activities curtailed. The first was purely a matter of trade competition. Official, state-sanctioned medical practitioners stood to gain financially if they could drive popular healers out of business through sustained Holy Office persecution. True, members of the lower social orders were generally not willing, let alone able, to pay the rates professional licensed healers charged for their services but, for a certain level of medical practitioner – country barbers, blood-letters and surgeons – there was a promising trade to be absorbed if rustics could be weaned away from their traditional cunning men and women. Further, licensed conventional healers at all levels of the profession stood to improve their strategic position as health care providers if they could discredit popular healing methods in the eyes of the general public. Beginning around the turn of the eighteenth century, then, licensed medical practitioners in Portugal lost their willingness to live with the contradiction of two separate, unequal, methodologically incompatible healing traditions in their country. Using their positions of influence within the Holy Office, they embarked on a program of systematic repression of magical healing, thereby promoting rationalized medicine at a time when other avenues to bring Enlightenment reforms to the medical profession in Portugal were closed.

Over the past quarter century, scholars writing mainly in Portuguese and English have succeeded in raising the historical profile of the early modern Lusophone world, providing colleagues and students with a better appreciation of the importance of the Portuguese as global disseminators of medical and botanical knowledge. Historians of two apparently disparate subjects – medicine and the Inquisition – are developing a clearer understanding of the wide social influence that members of the medical profession exercised, and their fundamental role in an imperial context as controllers and conduits of information about healing resources in the natural world, or about the commercial potential of those resources. As instruments of colonial policy, medical practitioners did their part to keep the limited Portuguese human resources healthy and fit for duty, to carry out the strategic aims of the empire. Their work within the Holy Office of the Inquisition was of a more limited scope, but no less important for the efficient functioning of the institution.

The surprising convergence of these two story lines makes for fascinating reading, but there is much left to consider. Opportunities for creative investigation exist in a number of areas: studies that specifically explore dimensions of race and gender; in-depth biographies of salient physicians who were credentialed as *familiars*; a detailed survey of the socio-economic backgrounds of licensed medical practitioners who worked for the Holy Office; and comparative studies that examine these dynamics in other European countries or in overseas colonial regions. There is no lack of future research possibilities regarding medicine and the Inquisition in the early modern world. We hope that the studies contained in this volume will inspire the next generation of scholars, who will make us richer for their efforts.

Index

Printed in the United States
By Bookmasters